Ruthless Winnicott

Ruthless Winnicott is an extended exploration of the role of ruthlessness in psychic development. That survival is of no use unless it is preceded by a ruthless attack is one of D. W. Winnicott's most resonant paradoxes. The book links this with the search for subjective freedom for those traumatized by colonialism, and in doing so draws on the work of Algerian psychiatrist and revolutionary psychoanalytic thinker Frantz Fanon.

Sally Swartz examines essential pieces of Winnicott's work on ruthlessness as central to the emergence of concern for the Other. She illustrates, with clinical examples, ways in which the ruthless use of the psychoanalytic psychotherapeutic space allows the patient either to enter fully into a process that allows growth, or to defend ruthlessly against the anxieties provoked by psychic change. *Ruthless Winnicott* also maps decolonial challenges to psychoanalytic theory, and the role of ruthlessness in protest movements demanding radical subjective change. Swartz's exploration of ruthlessness as both zest and defence in individual development and in protest movements illuminates processes of psychological collision and change. It traces links between individual trauma and collective turbulence, and maps ways in which ruthlessness is essential to subjective change.

Ruthless Winnicott will be of great interest to psychoanalysts and psychoanalytic psychotherapists, as well as scholars of colonialism, decolonization and post-colonialism.

Sally Swartz, PhD, is a psychoanalytic psychotherapist and academic, teaching, supervising and practising in Cape Town, South Africa. She has an enduring interest in the traumatic effects of colonialism, which was the subject of her monograph, *Homeless Wanderers: Movement and Mental Illness in the Cape Colony in the Nineteenth Century* (2015). *Ruthless Winnicott* brings together her interest in the history of colonialism in South Africa, psychoanalytic psychotherapy and the decolonial turn.

Ruthless Winnicott

The Role of Ruthlessness in Psychoanalysis and Political Protest

Sally Swartz

Routledge
Taylor & Francis Group
LONDON AND NEW YORK

First published 2019
by Routledge
2 Park Square, Milton Park, Abingdon, Oxon OX14 4RN

and by Routledge
711 Third Avenue, New York, NY 10017

Routledge is an imprint of the Taylor & Francis Group, an informa business

British Library Cataloguing in Publication Data
A catalogue record for this book is available from the British Library

Library of Congress Cataloging in Publication Data
A catalog record has been requested for this book

ISBN: 978-1-138-34548-5 (hbk)
ISBN: 978-1-138-34848-6 (pbk)
ISBN: 978-0-429-43663-5 (ebk)

Typeset in Times New Roman
by Swales & Willis Ltd, Exeter, Devon, UK

Contents

Acknowledgements

I have benefited deeply, over many years, from warm encouragement and generous engagement with colleagues in the International Association for Relational Psychoanalysis and Psychotherapy (IARPP) and the International Association for Psychoanalytic Self Psychology (IAPSP). Visits by members of both organizations to South Africa after the transition to democracy offered a rich source of learning. I have also been gifted with the opportunity to present some of my work at conferences hosted by both organizations and by the Training and Research in Intersubjective Self Psychology Foundation (TRISP). Without these presentations, and the discussions with which they were surrounded, I would not have written this book. I am especially grateful because of the many ways in which I was given the freedom to be creative and to be myself in these spaces, and was never asked to inhabit an uncomfortable diasporic or colonial identity. This was the beginning of a journey that I hope continues for many years to come. I would like to thank in particular Alejandro Ávila Espada, Jessica Benjamin, Margaret Black, Doris Brothers, Susi Federici-Nebbiosi, Victor Donas, Simone Drichel, Virginia Goldner, Uri Hadar, Stephen Hartman, Catherine Hicks, Hazel Ipp, Steven Knoblauch, Rina Lazar, Gianni Nebbiosi, Donna Orange, Eyal Rozmarin, Daud Saeed, Andrew Samuels, Lynne Segal and Chana Ullman for encounters at conferences, on panels and in colloquia that have shaped my thinking in profound ways. To have this collegial home to start from has been a wonderful thing.

There has also been a collegial community here in Cape Town, and my participation in it has been completely essential to my being able to think and write. This is the Cape Town Psychoanalytic Self Psychotherapy (CTPSP) group. This group, which embraces both self and relational theory and practice, has facilitated a steady flow of contact beyond our borders and kept a rigorous eye on our renewal of ourselves in terms of theory and technique. I am particularly indebted to colleagues with whom I taught and learned in various training course and seminars for psychoanalytic psychotherapists. Courses such as these make ruthless demands, and the benefits are magnificent.

I teach Masters Clinical Psychology students as they embark on their professional lives as psychotherapists. They are often working with patients who have suffered from multiple traumatic events and do not have the economic resources to seek mental healthcare in the private sector. I am very grateful to have been in these classes, and to have been given this space and time to reflect on the challenges we face in working with under-resourced and traumatized communities. A special thanks to the class of 2016, who cheerfully tolerated a period of everything in my mind circling back to Winnicott.

My first teacher and supervisor in psychoanalytic theory and practice was Fakhry Davids, now a psychoanalyst in London. His demand that I think deeply and systematically about the unconscious (and speak my mind!) set my course.

Valerie Sinason was a selfless visitor to Cape Town over many years, and her work in our courses and with colleagues about intellectual disability in particular taught me unforgettable lessons about respect and authenticity in the face of unbearable circumstances.

My friends and colleagues Jane Bennett, Stephen Bloch, Bev Dickman, Tony Frank, Louise Frankel, Margaret Orr, and Alison, Rebecca and Leslie Swartz read drafts of various chapters and provided me with feedback and encouragement to see this project through, even when I was inclined to put it aside. Steven Knoblauch's feedback on a chapter draft and his own new writing came at just the right moment. Tony Frank journeyed with me through teaching a short course on Winnicottian theory, and his support and guidance was wise and clear. I am also very grateful to Tony Frank and Ian Donald for our weekly peer supervision meetings, during which we get to play with psychoanalytic ideas in the safest of spaces.

Without my patients, none of this writing would have been possible. Each one has allowed me to see a little more clearly, a little further. Each has allowed us to organize a space in which we might become ruthless and compassionate together, a gift for which I am indebted to them. I am also very grateful to the staff and students with whom I had numerous conversations during the time of the protests. To have had this has changed most of how I think of myself in the world, and for this I am indebted to every one of my interlocutors. Particular thanks to Professor Sakhela Buhlungu, my dean during the time of the protests. His wisdom added immeasurably to what I was able to perceive. The psychotherapists at UCT's Student Wellness Centre were a formidable model of compassion and integrity through storms, and my conversations with them provided me with insight and friendship, for which I will always be deeply grateful.

Much of this book was drafted during a period of sabbatical leave from the University of Cape Town. My warm thanks to colleagues who covered my duties during that time. To my friends and family who made this writing retreat quiet during the day, but firmly connected to social spaces in the evenings and on weekends, thank you for keeping me on relatively dry land. To Stephen Bloch, Barbara Brookes, Bev Dickman, Paula Ensor, Tony Frank, Janet and Megan Grace, Gordon Inggs, Nan Loveridge, Anastasia Maw and Arddy Mossop in particular, thank you for your presence, and for knowing the inside of a writer.

My partner Margaret Orr's creative and loving presence during this time has carried me through many moments of self-doubt. Her belief in my resourcefulness has shaped profoundly my access to voice.

My daughters Alison and Rebecca Swartz honour me always by trusting me with their ruthlessness. They also trust themselves with mine, and together we never doubt our survival. At critical moments, Alison gave me an invaluable perspective on my central argument from a disciplinary space different to my own. There has been a precious resource in Rebecca and I supporting each other as we have both laboured over book projects. My daughters' writing, scholarly knowledge, curious reading of my work, and sharing of meals, socks, jerseys and holidays have all been woven into my writing, and made it a much sturdier thing. I wrote because I needed to try to make meaning of many experiences, but this act of writing is very small in comparison to their meaning in my life.

Introduction

Ruthless Winnicott and the decolonial project

Every time I reread a piece of Winnicott's writing, I find myself mulling over a new idea. This is not only about finding – always with gratitude – that something creative has been set in motion inside myself. It is also as if I have been freed to discover new textures and meanings in Winnicott's layered and enigmatic writing. That reading and rereading Winnicott is a creative joy has been powerfully explicated in Thomas Ogden's (2012) compelling account of the ways in which, as readers, we also write. This captures perfectly a Winnicottian appreciation of the significance of potential space and play. I feel indebted to Winnicott for writing in ways that allow reverie and provoke creativity, and to Ogden too, for his poetic rendition of the opportunity that has been put in our way.

Paradoxically, being struck by the originality of Winnicott's writing has everything to do with the way in which he constantly assumes familiarity. For example, when writing for a psychoanalytic audience, he assumes a canon, a genealogy of psychoanalytic ideas that he himself takes for granted and assumes is equally well known to his readers. When addressing parents and caregivers, he builds an argument around a host of instantly recognizable daily experiences of holding, feeding or playing with a child. There is also a comfortable familiarity in his tone that reverts frequently to the colloquial, his insistence on simple sentences and the charm of his humour. When he writes, "Some say: unanalysable, and throw up the sponge," or "The idea is sometimes put forward: of course everyone wants to regress; regression is a picnic; we must stop our patients from regression; or, Winnicott likes or invites his patients to regress," we have left behind the habitual solemnity of scientific papers. We are invited not only to join him in his gentle mockery of himself and others, but to hear them in conversations that have happened, and will certainly happen again (Winnicott, 2002, pp. 290–291). In the retention of rhythms of a paper being delivered to a live, breathing audience, he invites his readers to answer with sentences of their own. That this audience will be "reliable" in the sense of allowing itself to become preoccupied with what he has to say is also taken for granted. Perhaps his enduring popularity lies in his translation of the mysteries of internal worlds, tumultuous, violent, quiescent or joyful, into the observably ordinary; perhaps in the playful reciprocity between himself as writer/speaker and his readers. All this is familiar ground and constitutes the texture of a loved and well-used Winnicott, often idealized (Slochower, 2011), but also a psychoanalyst whose work has fed as richly into theoretical developments in psychoanalysis as its application in a wide range of mental health settings (Eigen, 2004, 2012).

This collection of essays is structured around one of Winnicott's words about non-compliance that has carried resonance for me (Newman, 1995). It is the word "ruthless," and in my exploration of it I have discovered my version of Winnicott. I believe that just as it is with his writing, this will contain much that is familiar, as it is a restating both of Winnicott and the psychoanalytic scholars who have written extensively about his work. I hope that my Winnicott creates the possibilities of new readings and writings, just as they have been created for me.

I first approached the idea of ruthlessness as it appears in Winnicott's writing as just that: an idea that he was treating with his usual kind and familiar common sense. As I wrote my way into the heart of the matter, the involvement of ruthlessness in originality, creativity and healing, I have come to respect deeply Winnicott's own ruthlessness, which he shows in the following ways. He demands the utmost commitment and presence from his readers. He insists on the creative potential of us all. He is unwavering in his focus on the tumult of early anxieties. He does not shy away from the frequently appalling compromises that are made in accommodating to uncaring or impinging environments. He continually reminds his readers of the suffering involved in seeking a reconnection with an authentic self. He does not spare either the psychoanalytic profession or himself the blunt examination of what it means to commit to the rigours of work on this interface between self and society.

The unconscious is ruthless in its insistence on its needs, its desire, its determination to be heard in symbol or symptom despite the agility of defences ranged against it. From its inception, psychoanalysis was of necessity ruthless in the terrain it covered. If Winnicott is to be described as ruthless, he is in good psychoanalytic company. There is nonetheless a unique way in which he performs ruthlessness. He proclaims the centrality of surviving ruthlessness to achieve the satisfactory relinquishment of omnipotence. He talks in a matter-of-fact tone about destroying the object, and then, discovering it alive, loving its new shape. He makes us all accountable to the ways in which we manage our survival of this destruction. He makes clear, too, that ruthlessness is a quality of vigour arising from a self making a demand, as well as the steady receipt of the ruthless attack without collapse into compliance or retaliation. There is sorrowing and triumph, failure, terror and periods of quiet regrouping. That it is momentous is never in doubt, but what ensures survival in the long run is this non-negotiable quality of personal accountability or presence. The paradoxical idea with which this book is concerned is trust that ruthlessness might be used in the service of entering reality with compassion. It has a constant focus on what this demands, both of those delivering a ruthless demand and those receiving it. To think about ruthlessness therefore requires that we also think about the nature of authenticity, recognition and of intersubjectivity itself.

This is well-trodden psychoanalytic territory, and in the first essays of the collection I am working with these familiar ideas with the aim of creating a particular slant of light, a focus on the quality of ruthlessness that accompanies the start of a cycle that leads through object relating to object usage, through muddle between inner and outer, projection and the real, into the creation of separate subjecthood. Here, I refer to the points at which the flow of projections gives way to periods of being able to see oneself from the outside in, and the object-becoming-other from the inside out.

The focus on ruthlessness in inner worlds is the necessary point of departure to two further centres of exploration illuminated by my particular slant of light. Winnicott reserved his use of the term "ruthless" to refer to the necessary zestful demand that a need be met. I am interested in other forms of ruthlessness, too, those designed to prevent impingements on the self. While these are well described as defensive strategies or character organizations, it is with their ruthless quality (and therefore their attack on intersubjective connection) that I am particularly concerned. I begin the book in Chapter 1 with my reading of Winnicott on ruthlessness in the service of zestful demand, and then elaborate on a number of clinical examples in which there are ruthless defences against connection. In Chapters 2 and 3, I look in detail at two kinds of ruthless defence: the ruthless coercion of the psychoanalytic situation through idealization, and then the ruthlessness of the peeping self, who thieves pieces of the therapy situation for private contemplation. These three chapters rehearse basic aspects of the theory I then apply to situations beyond individual psychoanalytic psychotherapy. They are also the necessary point of origin to which later sections inevitably return.

Second, I am interested in ruthlessness as it is lived through protest movements. The power of protests to disrupt ordinary routine, to destroy and demand recognition, is a form of ruthlessness. Focusing on it leads to two other avenues of exploration. There is the interface between the ruthless group, and the individuals using or being used ruthlessly by them, with the concomitant potential for destruction, trauma and renewal. Then there is the ability of protest movements to affect consciousness beyond participating individuals. That they are capable of changing public opinion is not in doubt. My interest is in the ways ruthless demands of protests groups might cause, over time, a shift in the way groups of individuals might experience themselves as actors and agents in time and space. These explorations are indebted to the work of many writing about the interface between individuals and the collective, but to the work of Jessica Benjamin (2017), Frantz Fanon (2004), Donna Orange (2008) and Joyce Slochower (2011) in particular.

The shift from object relating to object usage might be imagined as one in which the internal world is decolonized from the tyranny of both omnipotent control and persecution. Running through the book is this thread: to demand ruthlessly recognition from the other and freedom from internal objects by which one is held hostage is a decolonial project. Colonialism causes intersubjective damage, but also interpenetration, with the colonized and the colonizers defining each other's inner as well as outer worlds (Fanon, 1986, 2004). The decolonial movement involves a ruthless redefinition of consciousness, through destruction to a newly established, uncolonized landscape.

The second section of the book turns therefore to protest movements as an instance of ruthlessness. My own experience of the demand for decolonization at South African universities has felt simultaneously unique, as we do battle with the traumatic legacies and ongoing iterations of colonialism and apartheid, and deeply resonant, with protests in other parts of the globe. The #RhodesMustFall movement in South Africa lit a similar set of protests in Britain, most notably at Oxford University. These protests resonate with those about Confederate monuments across the United States precipitating debates about representations of history and memory, and the injuries caused by unthinking celebration of oppressive past leaders. The #BlackLivesMatter and #MeToo movements have their own permutations and a strong following in South Africa. And then there are all the rallies and fights for political, environmental and economic survival, marches against corruption, pleas for voices to be heard on gun violence, refugees, health provision and disability, and addiction that echo across continents, shaping themselves to particular contestations and deafness wherever they are found. In a world of instant communication through social media, protest movements speaking about injustices everywhere have wings and will fly. This gives psychoanalytic thinkers and writers a new responsibility: to describe the connections between social and unconscious terrors and rage; to think about the links between individual dynamics and those of groups or organizations; and to begin to imagine what it is that a protest movement might be expected to achieve, given the complicated intersections of class, race, sexuality and gender oppressions, the operations of privilege, and the endless propensity for histories to repeat.

In the second section of this book, I am using the South African university protests, as I experienced and thought about them, to think about these issues. Chapter 4 focuses on the link between individual trauma and organizational turbulence, and suggests that settings – rules, buildings and committee structures – have a containing function during periods of ruthless destruction. In Chapter 5, I pursue some of the ways in which the decolonial project demands not just a shift from object relating to object usage, but more radically to a new form of consciousness that heals double consciousness and the necessity for masks. I use the theories of Winnicott and Fanon in dialogue to explore this theme. Chapter 6 asks questions about representation, art, adornment and collective memory in periods of decoloniality. It has the removal of the statue of Cecil John Rhodes as its central focus. Chapter 7 describes shifts in consciousness, brought about by ruthless conflict, in people not directly involved in struggle, but nonetheless deeply affected by it. The book ends by using the experiences described in the book to consider the links between psychoanalysis and colonialism, to imagine decolonizing psychoanalysis as a project for our futures.

I have been aware, throughout my writing, of questions of authority and permissions to have access to voice. I am in what once was a psychoanalytic diaspora, without easy access to psychoanalytic training, frequent seminar programmes or regular presentations with internationally recognized psychoanalysts. We are still working through this legacy. Just as I would not therefore assume any kind of psychoanalytic authority, so too I do not presume to speak for protesters or protest movements. I am not even sure of the legitimacy of claiming the privilege of calling myself a witness, an issue I speak to the book's second section. There can be nothing more colonial than this internal struggle, and certainly little more ruthless than my being determined to have a say. My hope is that this statement of mine about a gathering together of bits and pieces of experience garnered over a tumultuous time will contribute to debate and creative readings far beyond my own imaginings.

Notes on patient confidentiality, clinical vignettes and terminology

I have illustrated my argument throughout this collection of essays with examples drawn from my experience as both an academic affected by student protest movements and as a psychoanalytic psychotherapist and supervisor. As always, patient confidentiality is a significant ethical wrestle for practitioner-writers. Clinical illustrations must be true if they are to be an honest accounting; they are not a work of fiction, but are not necessarily factual. They must be disguised in ways that maintain rigorously a relation to a truth, and yet maintain patients' rights to have their treatment kept vigilantly from all but professionally permitted readers. I have used a number of ways to protect the identities of those whose experiences I describe. I leave out all extraneous detail that might lead to their identification as a first and most fundamental step. I use disguise primarily in this way: I substitute an essential detail for another that is generically akin to it, in this way honouring my commitment to my account being true. So, for example, where my account calls for me to name a patient's career, I am careful to ascribe one that places him or her in a setting that would, in all important respects, share the qualities of the actual career being shared in the therapy. I do the same for leisure activities. I occasionally change the number and gender of a patient's siblings or children, but as this might affect the dynamics being described I have done this only when I have been sure that the integrity of my account is being maintained. There are times, especially in Chapter 1, where I have used composite vignettes, drawn from many years of clinical experience; in this case, disguise of an individual is not necessary. I will indicate in the text where I have done this. I have checked with those from whom I receive supervision, and those to whom I have given supervision on particular therapies, that my disguises are robust and also witness to truth.

Of course, readers have no way to verify my commitment to giving an honest account except their own sense of the coherence of the argument, its fit with the theory, and its affective resonance with their own range of social, political and clinical experience. I believe this to be a deeply rigorous test.

The literature on which these essays draws is psychoanalytic, and frequently assumes psychoanalysis as the activity to which the theory applies. As psychoanalysis has evolved both practically and theoretically, it is increasingly common to find references to face-to-face, once- or twice-a-week therapies in this literature.

These essays assume this form of engagement. My practice in South Africa is as a psychoanalytic psychotherapist. The literature I quote often refers to "the analyst," and I have preserved this where the term is used directly, but have used the term "therapist" in all other instances. By "therapist," I refer specifically to "psychoanalytic psychotherapist" throughout.

References

Benjamin, J. (2017). *Beyond doer and done to: Recognition theory, intersubjectivity and the third.* Routledge.

Eigen, M. (2004). *Psychic deadness*. Karnac.

Eigen, M. (2012). On Winnicott's clinical innovations in the analysis of adults. *The International Journal of Psychoanalysis, 93*(6), 1449–1459.

Fanon, F. (1986). *Black skin, white masks.* Pluto Press.

Fanon, F. (2004). *The wretched of the earth.* Grove Press.

Newman, A. (1995). *Non-compliance in Winnicott's words*. Free Association Books.

Ogden, T. H. (2012). *Creative readings: Essays on seminal analytic works*. Routledge.

Orange, D. M. (2008). Recognition as: Intersubjective vulnerability in the psychoanalytic dialogue. *International Journal of Psychoanalytic Self Psychology, 3*(2), 178–194.

Slochower, J. (2011). Analytic idealizations and the disavowed: Winnicott, his patients, and us. *Psychoanalytic Dialogues, 21*(1), 3–21.

Winnicott, D. W. (2002). *Through paediatrics to psychoanalysis: Collected papers.* Karnac.

Chapter 1

We want to be eaten

In "The Depressive Position in Normal Development," Winnicott makes a simple statement about the analyst's position: "We want to be eaten, not magically introjected." He goes on: "There is no masochism in this. To be eaten is the wish and indeed the need of a mother at a very early stage in the care of an infant" (Winnicott, 2002, p. 276).[1] To be eaten is to provide food for growth, to allow for digestion and expulsion. This underwrites transformation and the possibility of seeking enlivenment beyond simple physical survival.

The opposite of being eaten is not to be taken in as food, but to be used as a charm against hunger, a temporary balm in the form of an idealized and potentially addictive presence. "We hate to become internalized good breasts in others, and to hear ourselves being advertised by those whose own inner chaos is being precariously held by the introjection of an idealized analyst" (Winnicott, 2002, p. 276). For an analyst or psychoanalytic psychotherapist to be "eaten, worn down, stolen from" by a ruthless patient, and to survive, opens the way for a new form of relatedness. As Winnicott describes in "Primitive Emotional Development," it creates externality, "puts the brakes on" – allows freedom from – the magical world of fantasy, hallucination; it creates two, where before there was one, and in the survival of both negotiation might begin (Winnicott, 2002, p. 153; for a rich exploration of negotiation specifically in relation to paradox, see also Pizer, 2013).

For the infant to eat in the way Winnicott describes demands ruthlessness, in the sense that it is pitiless, without concern for effects. To mistake the infant as intending ruthlessness is to attribute a capacity for relationality that belongs to a later stage of development. To be ruthless is also not simply to be pitiless; in its full-throated demand, and in its expression, it embodies a vigorous act of trust. It is shamelessly naked, exposing the rawness of need as it is felt.

In "Hate in the Countertransference," Winnicott talks of the infant treating the mother "as scum, an unpaid servant, a slave" (Winnicott, 2002, p. 201). Holding hatred "without doing anything about it," particularly without retaliating, requires in itself a form of ruthlessness, this time the mother's. Tolerance is too passive a word to describe the quality of survival to be summoned while being used ruthlessly. It requires putting much else aside. Strong feeling has to be both contained and kept alive. The infant cannot use an emotionally absent or overwhelmed or terrified mother ruthlessly. Total presence is essential to survival of both mother and infant as a unit, and this, Winnicott argues, is possible because there is joy just as deep and wide and engulfing as the state of being worn thin. When Winnicott states that this is not masochistic, he refers to the unit living through and surviving an arduous experience together, without abdication, abnegation of self or enslavement to pain. And then there will be times during which quiet and sensual pleasure has joyously been achieved.

Survival of ruthlessness creates the quality of "ruth," defined by the *Oxford English Dictionary* as "the quality of being compassionate; the feeling of sorrow for another." Ruth implies the capacity to see the other, to experience the other as separate from oneself. For Winnicott, this early experience of ruth is inextricable from the destructiveness: ruth is compassion specifically for the other used ruthlessly in the service of survival. It is a "queer kind of truth" (Winnicott, 1989, p. 91).

We want to be eaten. Patients who are able to use us ruthlessly come to therapy to feed and be fed, all in the service of reaching beyond withdrawal from or persecution by an internal world made too present by a failure to survive. Winnicott suggests that to offer ourselves for eating in this way demands that we put aside our own preoccupations and ways of experiencing time. We are being asked to dream our patients, even when their capacity to dream might be damaged (Eigen, 2001, p. 65; Ogden, 2014, pp. 2–13). They will plunge deep and take us with them. It requires what Eigen refers to as "an area of faith" (Eigen, 1981, p. 413), or what Ghent calls "surrender" (Ghent, 1990, p. 108).

Winnicott put the word "ruthless" to work in two different ways. One signals absence of concern, which developmentally has not yet made its appearance. In "Psychoanalysis and the Sense of Guilt," he writes, "In analysis one could say 'couldn't care less' gives way to guilt-feeling" (Winnicott, 1965, p. 24). He refers in this to demand that does not yet take account of its cost. This use of the term might best be translated as zest, wholeheartedness or vigour. But Winnicott talks also of something more than careless zest; aggression is also at play, and will remain so, even after the establishment of concern, and the ability to separate destructiveness in fantasy from attacks on the loved and surviving "environment mother" (Lucente, 1998; Winnicott, 1965, p. 183). In that he considers it to be instinctual, he has accurately been taken to task for "valorization of hate, ruthlessness, and destruction" (Orange, 2011, p. 168).

In the chapters that follow, I will keep alive both threads of Winnicott's definition of ruthlessness. I will make the argument that defensive ruthlessness has a quality quite different to vigour or zest or wholehearted surrender. On the one hand, there is the possibility of zestful surrender to the vulnerability of "unfreezing"; on the other, a determination to prevent unfreezing, and to attack the therapist for attempting it. This book is about many permutations of ruthlessness across the range of both its meanings. Failure of ruth is sometimes temporary, sometimes enduring, and carried into cycles of deadness, compliance, dissociation or attack.

Ruthless pursuit of survival is common to both preservation of the original failure and subsequent thinness of concern, but also, in the right context, a reach for a new beginning.

"Hullo object!" "I destroyed you." "I love you." The creation of externality

In "Hate in the Countertransference," Winnicott outlines a number of reasons why a mother hates her infant "from the word go." The infant is free of worry for the mother's safety, mental health, need for sleep or need for the baby's cooperation in representing her as competent to the outside world. Not only is there dependence; there is an innocent disregard for what might be needed to make her feel good about herself. "His excited love is cupboard love, so that having got what he wants he throws her away like orange peel . . . He is suspicious, refuses her good food, and makes her doubt herself, but eats well with his aunt" (Winnicott, 2002, p. 201).

This baby demands that needs be met, and as time is frozen the needs are always urgent. The baby makes demands that tax the mother beyond her capacity to hold herself and to keep her own needs in mind. She must turn to others to have awareness of her needs. She is a slave, but her servitude puts at bay thoughts of her baby as her owner, her sovereign. She *is*, in her state of slavery, and for a time, she is her baby's thoughts, and the baby's needs are hers. The baby must be innocent, too, of the feelings stirred in her: "At first he does not know what she does or what she sacrifices for him. Especially he cannot allow for her hate" (Winnicott, 2002, p. 201). In order to preserve this ruthless use of herself, she must protect the baby from the kinds of "coincidences" that might bring doubt, catastrophic for being too early to bear. These might include physical pain in her absence or turbulence inside the mother caused by her ongoing life, separate from the baby. In other words, the baby must be sheltered from the kinds of everyday events that might prevent the caregiver from providing for a fretful child needing a sleep or a feed.

Given the stakes, survival of both the mother and the baby through the stage of ruthless need is an achievement and a labour. For the baby, ruthlessness received and survived paves the way for psychic aliveness, a faith that physical and psychological needs, however extreme and frightening, will be seen and attended to. This in turn allows time to unfreeze, so that there is space to imagine a future time, minutes or hours away, in which the vortex will be still. Negotiation becomes a possibility.

For the mother or caregiver, fuddled by lack of sleep, afflicted by anxiety and guilt when the baby is handed over to someone else so that laundry or grocery shopping might be done, there is relief and fury that she herself is at stake, even though she sometimes feels that she is hanging on by a thread. Along the way, there are moments of quiet, smiles and babbling, skin-on-skin togetherness. Joy, then, is as extreme as despair once was. Remarkably, these jewelled moments of pleasure are sufficient to see the dark nights through.

For Winnicott, survival of ruthless demand in the mother/baby unit is not simply a matter of time passing. It is not mechanical, because it is predicated on overwhelming and disorganizing affect that threatens going-on-being for both. It is not mechanical, because it is fully alive, and insists that feelings be felt. It is essential that the experience is lived together (Ogden, 2012, p. 90; Winnicott, 2002, p. 152). The baby begins to take something about survival for granted: that there is a going-on-being to be surrendered to and relied upon. Time opens too for the mother: she begins to attach in a new way to herself. Her interests broaden. She reads the newspaper occasionally, and relishes an hour of shopping alone.

The baby is not yet able to conceive of caring about the mother's survival, so that attacks are not for the purpose of destruction, and yet Winnicott insists not only that destruction occurs, but that it must occur. Destroyed is the baby's omnipotent control of the mother, as the baby "has doubts about himself" (Winnicott, 2002, p. 201). Destroyed also is the merged mother, the always-there failing, supplying, surviving mother. The mother, having been destroyed over and over as she carries her infant through early need, lets go at last of two things: her belief in the permanence of the unit itself, and then her belief in herself as omnipotently in charge of her baby's thriving. After living ruthlessness together, neither mother nor baby will be the same again. Failures are at times devastating, and a source of great anxiety. How they are managed will be critical to everything that follows.

Attempts at repair, reconstitution of the emerging in-and-out subject/object, are rendered as ruth, concern. Repair becomes a lifelong task. Crucially, ruth and ruthlessness, with all the implicit destruction and recreation, assertion, demand, forgiveness and compassion, are more than simple developmental events. As they recur, they are what makes feeling alive possible.

Imagine a child, 3 years old. She has a set of tiny teacups made from acorn cups and dried halves of orange skin. With ferocious concentration, she makes tea for the family – water, a little sand instead of sugar, some aloe juice for flavour. She stirs each potion with great care. Enormously pleased with her creation, she offers a cup to each person: "A lovely cup of tea for you!" mimicking her father's voice. She watches closely to make sure that tea is taken. Here is a glorious mixture of ruthlessness and concern. Her potion must be swallowed; she commands this, and no fobbing off will do. There is doubt too: will her tea be enjoyed? And into this gesture of hospitality is poured her understanding of a whole ritual of give and take, feeding and eating. There is both ruthlessness in the demand and concern for its effects.

This is perhaps Winnicott's most resonant paradox, one that has been the source of important revisioning of object relations theory (Benjamin, 2017; Eigen, 2001; Ogden, 2012; Pizer, 2013; Slochower, 2013). Survival is of no use unless it is preceded by a ruthless attack, an imagined destruction. It does far more than underwrite survivability itself. A death allows a recurring rebirth, and a pair where once there was one. It creates space between mother and baby, builds the capacity to experience a separate self, to use aloneness as a freedom, and to entertain murderous thoughts without assuming they will actually kill. Survival, happening as a result of destruction, and in cycles, constitutes the self as separate from the other, constructs point of view (what I see is not what you see), and begins to scaffold tolerance of ambiguity and contradiction. It sorts out the muddle between the baby's spontaneous gesture and the mother's receiving of it: from now on, the baby has a new sense of ownership of what comes from within. "Projective mechanisms assist in the act of *noticing what is there*, but are not *the reason why the object is there*" (Winnicott, 1969, p. 713, emphasis in original). This makes both love and mourning possible. Destruction is in the service of being able to feel fully alive, because external reality is reassuringly knowable, and puts "the brakes" on the terrifying world of fantasy and merger (Winnicott, 2002, p. 153). Ogden argues that the creation of externality is simultaneously the creation of the unconscious (Ogden, 2016, p. 1255). "Here fantasy begins for the individual" (Winnicott, 1969, p. 713). While object relating "can be described in terms of the subject as an isolate," object usage involves the object "being part of shared reality, not a bundle of projections. It is this, I think, that makes for the world of difference that exists between relating and usage" (Winnicott, 1969, p. 711).

Neither ruthlessness nor ruth is immutable or even solidly enduring over time.

There are two strands to be followed in exploring further the significance of ruthlessness in psychic life. One concerns the many permutations of ruthlessness in the individual for whom ruth, in balance with ruthlessness, is firmly established, and for whom guilt, mourning and compassion are all a possibility. The other is concerned with individuals in whom a capacity for negotiating externality and gathering together of bits and pieces in the face of destruction can never be taken for granted. Here, ruthlessness is predicated on survival of a self and object fusion, in the absence of a steady backdrop of externality. The role of aggression in both needs to be held in mind.

As illustration, those for whom ruth is a constant companion may be unseated by ruth itself. When there is overwhelming worry about or subjection to the fate of another, dissociation or self-protective withdrawal might come into play for a time. At the other extreme, those for whom pre-ruth is a way of remaining relatively free, consciously at least, of earliest agonies, acts of generosity and thoughtfulness sometimes occur, however sequestered or ringed around with defence or brittleness. I will be arguing that an awareness of movement in and out of states of ruthlessness and ruth, their relationship to achievement of object usage, and the meaning of each for an understanding of a patient's needs of the therapy is helpful for both diagnosis and treatment.

Muddles

The road from ruthlessness to ruth is not straightforward. It is possible to reconstruct through Winnicott's prolific descriptions of mother/baby units the multiple ways in which the process might be compromised (Winnicott, 1971, 1990). There is an important caveat, however: all mother/baby units experience some bumps and bruises. It is the pattern that matters, not bad hours or days taken singly. Winnicott begins from a place of assuming resilience, even as he imagines us into a world in which psychic survival cannot be taken for granted. In the idea of the "good enough" is of course the idea that ordinary failures are seldom catastrophic, so long as the steady pattern is one of satisfactory provision. What is good enough will vary from unit to unit, depending on a range of challenges to be faced. Against the stark backdrop of destructiveness and the onslaught of early emotional life, the assumption of resilience is vested in two places: the mother's "primary maternal preoccupation," a kind of illness that allows fierce protectiveness of the doubly dependent new person being hatched, and in the infant's own will to live (Winnicott, 2002, pp. 302–303).

There are several ways in which ruthlessness is rendered futile, and in that sense emptied of meaning. In cases of neglect, the baby's ruthless demand is unfelt, unheard or ignored, and crying itself may stop, as the baby drifts into psychic deadness or traumatic dissociation. But then there is the opposite. Continuous crying, with no periods of quiet satisfaction or pleasure, may cause the mother to feel that responding is futile. Over-exact anticipation of the baby's every need also renders ruthlessness futile, as there is no space for the need to be experienced at all. Ruthlessness may also become distorted when the baby's need is persistently misinterpreted: hunger as cold, cold as tiredness, and so on. Fobbing off the baby by responding to a need imagined by the mother but not attuned to the baby's state carries the danger of folding the baby into compliance or despair. It brings the danger of muddling profoundly links between psyche and soma as the baby begins to associate hunger with temperature, or food with feeling cold or wet.

Too deep a resonance with the baby's affective state also carries dangers. By receiving the baby's terror with terror of her own, the mirroring mother amplifies her ruthless baby's ocean of affect. The mother is alive, and revisiting her own baby terror; despite aliveness, survival is constantly in doubt. As Fonagy and his colleagues point out in the literature on attachment and mentalization, contingent affective responsiveness regulates through resonating with the general colouring of the baby's affect, without reproducing it in exact form (Allen et al., 2008; Fonagy, 2006, p. 68; Fonagy and Campbell, 2015, p. 236).

Further, if the mother is experienced as empty internally, or psychically dead, the baby gives up on lusty demands, because the response to them is drained of affect and devoid of spontaneity. Some mothers retaliate, matching the baby's ruthlessness with anything from a punishingly strict timetable to rough handling and anger. If this is the case, any expression of ruthlessness by the infant comes packaged with echoing fear. Some mothers are able to convince their babies that they are alive only when they are locked into tumult, with the between spaces disconnected and drifting into deadness. And finally, some come and go, getting it right some of the time, and temporarily convincing the baby to have faith. Then they become angry, go numb or disappear, casting everything into despair made worse by the hope of the hour before. In Winnicott's view, "The mother here has as part of her illness a need to cause and to maintain a muddle in those who are in contact with her" (Winnicott, 1965, p. 147).

How, then, does failure to carry the child over from early ruthlessness into ruth map on to demands that might materialize in adult treatments? The following sections will begin with a description of ruthlessness in psychoanalytic work used productively to carry the patient through from object relating to object usage. The chapter will then move on to describe defensive ruthlessness, as it might appear in a range in patient treatments. These are sketches only, using composite vignettes. Further theoretical and technical exploration, illustrated by case studies, follows in Chapters 2 and 3.

Ruthlessness in the service of change

I begin here by describing the quality of ruthlessness that signals not only its use in making the therapy a working space, but also the presence of ruth as a surrender to negotiation.

A woman comes for therapy at a time of difficulty in a long-term relationship with an imperious partner. In arguments with him, she becomes scared, muddled and then "shuts down." She then experiences herself as unable to think, and she withdraws both physically, by going for walks or going to sleep, and emotionally, by failing to be stirred into participating in the emotional storm gathering around her. This creates further conflict as her partner accuses her of retreating in order to avoid intimacy. Internally, she enters a spiral of self-blame, partly accepting her partner's accusations and partly punishing herself for remaining in a relationship that is causing her increasing unhappiness.

She has warm friendships, a successful career in business, and is deeply trusted by colleagues, with no immediate difficulties apart from the turbulence in her relationship. However, she is beginning to feel a resentment and a numbness that blocks her access to a sense of liveliness. She has a history of being fathered by an autocratic man who demanded her absolute acquiescence, and who bullied her in a vitriolic way if she showed independent opinions. The links between the tumult in her relationship and her father's style, her tendency to be compliant, and her fear, leading to dissociation, quickly become the focus of the therapy.

In this therapy, the setting is taken for granted, and boundaries are easily adhered to. She warns early on that she does not trust easily, and yet she offers material that provokes deep discussion. She opens layers of thoughts articulately, and in ways that lend themselves to linking, and that demand a sinking into connection. This comes with a sensation of being intruded upon, rearranged, muddled up inside. There are times when an interpretation is experienced as a demand for compliance, or an imperious judgement of her attempts to discover her own needs. She then describes herself as becoming "fuzzy," and struggles to follow the thread of her narrative. She has to stop talking and stare out of the window. She is readily aware in these times of feeling resentful towards her therapist for unsettling her in ways that she experiences as profound.

She is ruthless in bringing herself through in the therapy, and in allowing the full significance of a past pattern of object relating to flow through it. She has ruth in collecting herself and her bits and pieces at the end of each session.

This is a patient able to engage, surrender to the heady ebb and flow of strong feeling, relish discovery, and entertain hateful feelings, vigour in battle and gratitude for the process of change. Eigen describes "experiencing which is undertaken with one's whole being, all out, 'with all one's heart, with all one's soul, and with all one's might'" (Eigen, 1981, p. 413). Faith in the process is mostly preserved. Here, the patient notices many things about the therapist – her interests, tired days, stiff back, change in wardrobe – but is able to put aside ruth (here specifically guilt, or a wish to be a good and undemanding patient) in order to access her own dream, and to insist that she and her therapist dream together (Ogden, 2014).

Ruth may not be conscious, and is therefore not consciously put aside; it is at play, however, in a number of ways. It is present in the patient's capacity to work with rupture and repair, which always implies the possibility of forgiving and moving on (Lachmann and Beebe, 2013). Ruth also makes space for some of the therapist's needs, accommodating her occasional slide into jargon, say, or a theoretical lecture or temporary enthusiasms. She accommodates the therapist's language, even its quaint bits of technical language, which she takes on as her own. She shapes herself in this respect to the therapist's style. Ruth moderates ruthlessness to the extent that it contains the demands of dependence to the parameters of the treatment itself. This patient has the capacity to be alone (Winnicott, 1965), to enter her own reverie (Ogden, 1997), follow her thoughts and also to play. The therapist is included, but also trusted not to impinge on the interplay of projection and externality.

For her part, the therapist uses interpretation with tact. Ruthlessness contained by ruth in this way has integrity and momentum; the therapist's task is to hold the setting. Winnicott cautioned against interfering with process by unneeded interpretation:

> It appals me to think how much deep change I have prevented or delayed in patients in a certain classification category by my personal need to interpret. If only we can wait, the patient arrives at understanding creatively and with immense joy, and I now enjoy this joy more than I used to enjoy the sense of having been clever. I think I interpret mainly to let the patient know the limits of my understanding.
>
> (Winnicott, 1969, p. 711)

Ruthlessness for Winnicott belongs partly to a time before ruth makes its appearance, and is necessary for survival, insofar as it enables destruction, and then guilt, mourning, reparation and love. So, in the description of this healthy ruthlessness, where is the destruction? Is survival at stake at all?

The answer to this lies in several directions. Within the therapy room, there is regression of the benign sort Winnicott describes in "Metapsychological and Clinical Aspects of Regression within the Psycho-Analytical Set-Up." This is specifically regression to a state of dependence on the treatment, the room, and the therapist that repeats a successful holding in the early environment

(Winnicott, 2002, p. 283). It places an ethical responsibility upon the therapist that is not open for negotiation. It demands, ruthlessly, the therapist's capacity to become "preoccupied with the patient," "being alive, breathing." The therapist must be "much more reliable than people are in ordinary life." All this is in the realm of the ruthless. The survival of the therapist is therefore at stake. Moreover, the regression itself is not "a picnic," and requires surrender, and at least at the outset is courageous; this, too, implies survival (Winnicott, 2002, p. 285).

Second, the useful suffering of a benign regression is best served by a free play of talk, reverie, dreams and feeling (for a description of "useless suffering," see Eigen, 2004, p. xv). These inevitably lead the patient to make with the therapist the kind of interaction that will open the parts of the past that need to be aired. Whether one casts this in the language of enactment (Bromberg, 2013; Stern, 2013), internal working models and attachment blueprints (Mitchell, 2014; Wallin, 2007) or transference (Racker, 2012), there is agreement broadly that the therapist will be used at least partly to bring to the situation painful past experience. The "blooming, buzzing confusion" (James, 2013), of interplay, the muddle of inside/outside, the object and the environment, is a feature of ruthlessness, of object relating, as opposed to object use. And the working through *destroys* that mingling, so that repair and gratitude will survive. As Ghent puts it:

> One might imagine the subject saying to the object, "I went all out, completely vulnerable, in the faith [or surrender] that someone was out there – and it turned out to be true, as I could only have known by destroying you with all my might, and yet here you are. I love you."
>
> (Ghent, 1990, p. 108)

His majesty and the mouse – the ruthlessness of entitlement and compliance

I turn now to ruthlessness of another sort, the kind that invokes useless rather than useful suffering (Eigen, 2004), or that feeds directly into repetition of traumatic patterns of relating. I will describe two ends of a continuum, with obliviousness at one end and vigilant obedience to a set of rigid rules at the other.

There is ruthlessness in the entitled patient, who commands the space of the therapy room and obscures the living presence of the therapist. This is someone startled to find she cannot dictate the timing or length of sessions, or set the dates of the therapist's vacation. She cannot imagine a busy schedule involving other patients, just as she cannot imagine her therapist being unavailable for her after-hours calls.

There are a number of traumatic routes to a state of mind in which entitlement features heavily, and these include both neglect at one end of the scale and magical fulfilment of every wish or need at the other. As Kohut (1971) has convincingly demonstrated, underlying a grandiose self-presentation is a fragile foundation to a sense of self. Of critical importance is the difference between the ruthless and persistent erasure of the other to be found in states of entitlement, and the ruthless exploitation of the therapy situation described in the previous section. In the latter, negotiation is possible; object usage enables a therapeutic frame, with its agreed-upon boundaries and rules, to be in place. There is an exchange of affect, and an experience is lived together, repeated, dreamed and reflected on. For the entitled patient, this is only sometimes possible.

Omnipotence is evident in the way that the frame is subjected to magical thinking. So, for example, a patient magically reduces the time it takes him to reach his therapist's office in fantasy, omnipotently clearing the roads of traffic, and not doubting the appearance of a parking space just outside the building. Arriving for his session late and unruffled, and commenting with irritation on the traffic he did not expect, he settles into the chair and begins the session with a number of questions about the therapist's views on political events, requiring her to parry, and to try to make links with what she knows about the patient's underlying concerns, to collect him into the analytic work. He smiles knowingly, and suggests ways she might think about the political situation. He assures her that this will be helpful for her and her patients. Twenty minutes into the 50-minute hour, he turns to himself, and in leisurely detail describes what he would like to discuss in the session.

The session, of course, comes to an end unmagically, and without much having been done. There has been no time for the therapist to explore or comment. More seriously, denigration, both implicit and explicit, and a quality in the ruthlessness itself, which carries aggression rather than vigour, short-circuits the therapist's thinking. She wonders why this patient continues to come, and ruminates uncomfortably about the ways in which she has been complicit with a space in which full engagement is sabotaged.

This kind of ruthless control of the session prevents the possibility of a relational exchange. As coercive shaping of the encounter is designed unconsciously to obliterate the alive presence of the other, there can be no connection. In this, there is a ruthless defence against being confronted with externality, a multiplicity of views, potential attunement failure and independent-mindedness. All of these are potentially frightening as they carry overwhelming anxiety about an interruption in going-on-being, through disappointment, abandonment or aggression. There is nonetheless a feeding that takes place in the therapy session, but it involves the patient feeding himself, since "feeding from an other-than-me source" is not yet possible (Winnicott, 1969, p. 712).

It is possible to suppose, therefore, that the patient's apparent commanding presence represents bits and pieces that have been gathered only as a way of forestalling dread; there is an illusion of cohesion that acts as a spell against disaster. It is possible to imagine here a baby for whom neglect or incursion, and survival despite this, was both a triumph and carried an unsteady sense of relief in the face of falling forever. It is also possible that here was a baby whose mother met need with hyper-vigilance, believing that even a moment of distress would precipitate calamity. For such a patient, the heart cannot be worn on the sleeve, and yet hiding altogether implies the disaster of not being found (Winnicott, 1965, p. 186).

Erasure of the therapist by the entitled patient has an odd counterpart in the patient who erases herself from the therapy situation, by presenting only what she believes to be acceptable to her therapist. She becomes a parrot, a mime, fending off the disaster of mismatch, and of negotiating towards mutuality (which she "knows" is not possible) by pitch-perfect performance. As Winnicott puts it, "the analysis goes with a swing" (Winnicott, 1989, p. 91). The frame is intact, except insofar as she monitors the ending time of the session herself, not wanting to overstay her welcome. She follows the rules diligently, scanning the environment anxiously for clues on how to behave in the room, when to use the tissues or the bathroom. She pays attention to the opening and closing of doors. Within the session, she busily weaves a collage like the ghost of a reverie, not her own bits and pieces, but rags garnered from the therapist's sentences, clues offered by interpretations or the therapist's apparent lively interest in certain strands of her history. There might be feelings in the room, but they are carefully managed so as not to worry, overwhelm or impose a demand on the therapist. In Winnicott's "Ego Distortion in Terms of True and False Self," he describes acting:

> There are those who can be themselves and who also can act, whereas there are others who can only act, and who are completely at a loss when not in a role, and when not being appreciated or applauded (acknowledged as existing).
> (Winnicott, 1965, p. 149)

Compliant patients can only act.

An entitled or grandiose patient takes command of the therapy time by treating the beginning and ending of sessions, in fantasy, as within his or her control. Attacks on the frame might include intrusive commentary on the room itself, or the insertion of topics garnered from the daily news. In comparison, sessions with the compliant patient are likely to begin and end exactly on time. The patient hands herself over to the frame in the sense of coming in and sitting still, perhaps in a way that suggests the impossibility of lounging or stretching. She might take a sip of a glass of water in a way that suggests polite use of a provision rather than thirst. The refusal to surrender to the space, to feel free enough to allow something spontaneous to emerge, is a ruthless defence against vulnerability.

She begins with the previous session:

> Remember you mentioned last week that I might take on too much because I am afraid of my boss's disapproval? Well yesterday, he asked me to do an extra four hours of tutoring with students. I said no! I can't do it this month!

She checks the therapist's response by glancing quickly at her face.

> I felt so pleased afterwards. I can say no! He was fine with it. He asked someone else! And I had a dream about closing the door on a woman wanting to come into my kitchen. I woke up thinking I am going to stop my co-workers from using my milk.

Here, there is compliance ironically with what has been discerned as the therapist's programme: not to comply. Even the unconscious seems to cooperate, producing a dream in which assertiveness apparently appears. It is difficult indeed to interpret this dream other than affirmatively; the suggestion that the patient is in fantasy shutting her therapist out of her kitchen, where she has milk entirely for herself, might well be met with puzzlement or withdrawal. For Winnicott, this is mimicry "of the True Self *as it would be if it had had existence*" (Winnicott, 1965, p. 146, emphasis in original).

The danger for this patient is the depletion experienced as a result of the strain of compliance. At some point, the outflow of energy preserving the object becomes so burdensome that an ending is sought, without the possibility of nourishment ever having been provided, apart from pieces stolen and examined privately.

There are a number of routes to this traumatized presentation: perhaps this patient has been met with overwhelming anxiety if she expressed need or came to understand that deviation from a prescribed pattern of behaving unleashed catastrophic affect. Regardless of the route, this patient, just like the entitled one, is ruthless in ruling out an exchange in which the spontaneous gesture might be made and received.

Ruthless independence

There is a kind of ruthlessness in patients who accomplish their own analysis, rendering the therapist extraneous, apart perhaps from delivering a setting. The patient brings dreams, associates to them in the session, but is ready too with an interpretation. For example, this is a person who might comment on a tearful moment in a meeting during the week, and then recounts the events as a repetition of family dinner table tension, doing the linking without the need for the therapist's thoughtful intervention.

Another example might be a patient who is thoroughly versed in psychoanalytic theory and technique, and who presents an inner world alongside a commentary on her hidden anxieties and defences, moments of rupture or misunderstanding, signs of dissociation or retaliatory remarks. These might be presented with rueful concern. The challenge in this is that while the inner world is presented with disarming richness, and the analysis of its meaning, as far as it goes, seems accurate, there is a fundamental avoidance of the kinds of ruthless engagement that might allow for destruction and relational reconstitution. In other words, there is no opportunity to test the boundaries of survival; going-on-being is invested solely in the patient's determination to live and to thrive on resources entirely generated from within. There is no surrender to the situation, no nod given to the area of faith of which Eigen speaks, and little spontaneity. Most importantly, the independent patient has neither capacity to be alone nor ability to use potential space for play: as Winnicott argues in "The Capacity to Be Alone," these both require an ability to move between, to enter reverie despite and because of the presence of another, to entertain another's imaginings, and to use the gap between to create rather than to present an already known world (Winnicott, 1965). The work is always already completed, and cannot be shared in the making; conclusions have been reached, the end result is signed off and filed. It may be shared as a gift or a punishment, a shy achievement for approbation, or a reminder of the therapist's incompetence. A comment on this as a feature of the treatment is simply an occasion for further independent work, and a more polished performance next time.

Ruthlessness takes the form of showing up, and making the therapist an audience to a performance apparently faultless and full of meaning, but leaving the therapist omnipotently controlled. In this situation, it is reasonable to wonder whether the work is indeed being done, and whether performing insight (for example) and sharing it as a fait accompli might take on the colouring of an alive sharing.

Here, there are two possibilities. It may happen that a patient maintains a secluded fantasy relationship with the therapist, even a thick dialogue that occurs internally between sessions. The "gift" of work done is reported, rather than shared, but nonetheless the therapist is kept apprised of developments, and if nimble may create opportunities for the spontaneous gesture to be brought and received. The outlook is less optimistic when the patient runs the treatment in two parts – a secret part, conducted alone, and a curated pseudo-analysis presented as if it is real. In "The Patient Who Is Difficult to Reach," Betty Joseph remarks that some "are in fact doing a great deal of acting" (Joseph, 1989, p. 164). It is a more difficult performance to carry through than one that is conveying work in an actual passage of time; it is full of placeholders and easily creeps into cliché and repetition, magpie material stolen from the nests of other birds.

As with the compliant patient, the therapist finds her own words taken over and given back, and a wish to be compliant might be a feature in both. The two kinds of colonization, however, serve fundamentally different purposes. One is a pathological accommodation in which object substitutes for self; the other is a sequestered self, rebellious, creative, stubborn, but always in disguise.

Its secrecy creates the risk of the therapist's disengagement, his or her own sense of uselessness leading to premature suggestion of terminating, or failure to appreciate ways in which this independence is not self-sustaining at all, but is invested in a world of regularity in time and setting.

This kind of ruthlessness may have come into being as a result of reward for competence and problem-solving in the world, in the absence of an effective holding of spontaneity. It may have come about through withdrawal from unreliable, volatile or mis-attuned mothers or a demanding, impinging environment. It does suggest a sequestered true self that becomes a source of initiative and soothing, but a self that fears an undressed encounter, except through false self-mediation.

The ruthlessness of the fussy eater

It is ruthless to refuse the therapist's every contribution, even when this is no more than a reflecting back of the patient's own words. Interpretations for this kind of patient are never quite right. It may be that they pick at their own sentences too, correcting word choice, trying to find something that matches precisely a thought or event. The corrections and corrections to corrections desiccate the conversation, and the living of an experience is reduced to approximations and proxies, a stumbling conversation in search of roots in meaning. This is like trying to feed a fussy or colicky baby, for whom food of any kind is an impingement. Ruthlessness takes the form of creating a witness to a process of starvation, always wondering if a change in this ingredient or that will allow something to be taken in. An extraordinary and valiant effort is needed, a testing and tortured path, in which the patient watches with puzzlement, disdain, scorn or even self-pity. The patient sometimes appears to be lost in a material world, the key to which is matching colours and ruling straight lines. It is a critical place, overseen by a squat superego, calling out wrongness, not of life itself (for that would be depression), but the wrongness of pleasure, connecting and creativity.

For example, a patient might describe a situation at home in which his wife criticizes him for his choice of words as he tells her about a moment of accomplishment of which he had been proud. It is described as a moment of failed communication between them, an attack, and yet he deflects the therapist's attempt to put into words the emotion stirred. "No," he says, "I was not deflated." "No, I did not feel angry." He tells how he withdraws in these circumstances, punctured; his wife calls him narcissistic, and this sets in train days of rumination about his personality, his lack of achievements in his career, his failure to encourage his children. The therapist makes a general comment about the moment in which he showed an important piece of himself to his wife and was met with a rebuff, with reverberations in his sense of self-esteem. He listens sceptically, and then remarks, "But she is right, I am narcissistic," and presents evidence of this. The therapist then comments on the orchestration of his self-attack with the wife's attack. At this hint of finding a therapeutic ally, he redoubles his self-attack, assuring the therapist that he is absent-minded, grumpy and impatient. As he speaks, he picks up a small piece of leaf lying on the carpet. He is dusting the setting, and the situation, off.

One imagines anxious or critical parents in this baby's failure to be carried over from ruthlessness to ruth. Difficulty with taking in and absorbing anything offered from the outside may have had its origins in routines of feeding in infancy. This might have been accompanied by physical experience that included pain or discomfort, or emotional experience of impatience or worry that mixed the sensation of allowing something in to become mixed with its immediate rejection. There is no expansiveness in this pitiless landscape.

It also seems possible to imagine a patient whose difficulty with absorbing the nourishment of the therapeutic space has arisen from a childhood world never suffused with emotional meaning. This is perhaps a way of coming into being that was confined to materiality: puzzles, blocks, to be built right – and built until right – towers not to be kicked over, but packed neatly in rows. Dealing with the realm of emotional connection is then a matter of puzzling over a foreign body, one that cannot be ordered, but must be isolated and ejected.

Of course, the enigma in this situation is that the patient has come with the hope of being fed, despite the ruthless rejection of the food on offer. The offer of food, and its rejection, becomes the proxy feeding, a repetition of never reaching a state of satiation.

Absent-mindedness

There is a paradox of ruthlessness in the absence of mind-mindedness that features in work with patients for whom dissociation or failure to achieve mindedness is a central feature. Therapy demands reflection (whether shared or not) and communication (whether in talk or silence); it is therefore in itself ruthless. The demand of the setting – showing up, thinking and communicating, sharing feeling, coming back to do it all again, week after week – is sufficiently anxiety-provoking to precipitate dissociation or incoherence in those vulnerable to either. Unless the ensuing dialogue is entirely irrelevant to the patient's difficulties, both form and content of each session must add to the burden of remaining both present and mindful. The paradox lies in the patient's inability to use the therapy in a ruthless way, either defensively, to wall out connection, or to reach through destruction (eating) to creation and survival. This is not to say that the quality of ruthlessness is absent. It becomes by default located in the setting, on the one hand, and in the therapist's ruthless pursuit of the vanishing mind, on the other.

For example, a patient whose every thought, every spontaneous gesture, was ridiculed by her envious father as she grew up managed her emotional life by losing her capacity to "think straight." With compromised memory and loss of a syntax of mind – logic, ability to link subject and object, to sequence events in time, to attribute causality appropriately, to connect a feeling with a either verb or noun – she flounders through an endless series of bewildering experiences intersected by black holes. In therapy, she brings an account of the events of a day, but this did not necessarily lead forwards or backwards, nor have any obvious connection to a knot to be unravelled, or a feeling to be amplified and turned over. At other times, she gives a tumbled, disjointed account of a worry or a dilemma, and time would be spent trying to unweave the tangle of delicate threads all in a ball. Always there would be a moment at which she would fall silent, cast on her own emptiness, panicking at point blank. She would then plead with her eyes for rescue, for something to be provided – anything: talk, the session's end, the offer of reassurance. In situations like these, the pressure on the therapist to fill in the blanks is propelled by versions of "primitive agonies" – going to pieces, falling forever, disorientation, mind and body split apart.

The dissociative patient defends against having a mind-syntax, remembering and linking, as a defence against the pain of having once thought or felt: there is an experience, whether formulated and buried or unformulated and captured in an affect-cloud. This differs from the person for whom neglect rather than attack was the cause of failure in capacity to think. For this patient, there has been enough bodily care to ensure physical survival, perhaps even orientation to the physical world, upside and downside. The absence is in vocabulary that ties time to the world, and both to reflection and feeling. Events become random, insecurely located between past, present and future, the plots of stories are thickets of contradiction, and feelings gather like iron filings on inconsequential magnets. For a patient struggling with mind in this way, arriving at therapy is in itself an achievement, for the purpose of talking is never to be taken for granted and may often feel unnecessary or futile. There is in this situation a ruthless demand on the therapist to construct a mind from the bits and pieces.

For example, a patient presents in the first instance as fragmented or scattered – there is no coherent narrative from the past or present, and there is a struggle to locate family members in their right order, or to track ordinary sequences in births, marriages and deaths. Quite soon, she reports that there is a pregnancy, as if it is not happening in her own body. It is denied a material existence in that there is no real appreciation of a foetus growing day by day. At the same time, there is an ongoing fantasy about seeking a termination of the pregnancy. The patient's husband, and only sexual partner, is not told of the pregnancy, which he wants very much. The therapist, faced with the drifting around the decision about the termination, feels increasingly impelled to draw attention to the fact of weeks going by, and opportunities for choice being foreclosed. Interventions about needing to decide whether to keep the pregnancy or not are made to no avail. Sessions are taken up or discarded in a chaotic way during this time. There is despair, but its link to the pregnancy remains unclear. In this way, the pregnancy happens to therapist and patient without planning, either to seek it or keep it, and it is nearly five months before the baby's father even becomes aware of it. The ruthlessness invested in this situation is that of management being needed: of the health of mother and baby in a quite practical way, and a nesting not being done, while the apparatus for bearing the unit in mind is isolated in the therapist's mind, and yet has no bearing, no traction or exchange of meaningful words.

Ruthless attack

A patient comes to therapy, and, apart from a worrying lack of cohesion in her presenting story, she is quirky, appealing and uses the initial sessions in an ordinary way. She hints at difficulties concentrating, and suicidal thoughts in her past. There is occasional drug abuse, and a romance with a man she describes as taking her into trance-like ecstatic states. There is a difficult relationship with a critical mother, who intrudes on her life in disruptive ways.

There comes a period during which an outer shell gives way to extreme vulnerability. She wails loudly in sessions, on and on, asking to be physically held. She throws a book. During vacations, she demands telephonic contact. She writes novel-length letters about her despair at this therapy-love. There are times of paranoid thinking mixed with deep depression. She is dependent on the therapy but tortured by it. Her family is stirred up by her complaints and threatens the therapist with a malpractice suit. Hospital and psychiatric medication are always in the wings. The suffering is endless, useless and awful.

This malignant regression was perhaps inevitable, and was certainly predictable from the earliest sessions. It demonstrates a kind of rule-breaking, frame-destroying emotional violence precipitated by the kind of care suggested by the setting: the quiet, the preoccupied attention, the regularity, the alive and listening therapist. Its "malignancy" rests in its relentless repetition of the original failure, along with its emotional storms, often inaccessible to languaging. It does not necessarily imply that it is inaccessible to help or soothing; instead, the focus of attention shifts from talk to the setting itself, frequency of contact, and strategies for affect regulation and awareness of mental states (Fonagy, 2000; Winnicott, 2002).

Ruthless states such as these are brought about by disintegration and frantic attempts to get the therapist to gather the bits and pieces together. The suffering implied in demands seems to give voice to "primitive agonies" lived over and over, and they undo ordinary therapeutic care. In Winnicott's view, for these patients the "personal structure is not yet securely founded." As a consequence of this, "the accent is more surely on management, and sometimes over long periods with these patients ordinary analytic work has to be in abeyance, management being the whole thing." By this, he means "the mother actually holding the infant" (Winnicott, 2002, p. 279; for detailed discussion of the implications of "holding," see Slochower, 2013).

Not all ruthlessness associated with emotionally violent object relating is this present or so obviously in need of direct management. Some is subtle or out of reach, ranging from cruel or sarcastic comments, through to the therapist being used as a witness to violence in or outside of the therapy. This might consist, for example, of reported abuse of elders, children or partners, and self-attack in the form of refusing food, drug and alcohol abuse, and suicide threats, attempts and cutting. As witness, the therapist is sometimes in bondage, poised between action that will preserve the therapeutic dialogue and obligation to be ruthless herself, through an out-of-therapy intervention such as a hospital admission or referral to another agency. Of course, there is sometimes a third way, a delicate choice of words, a suggestion or decision that preserves the therapy while at the same time setting clear behavioural parameters.

Both forms of ruthlessness, overt and indirect, are linked with coercion: prisoners are taken, and hostage negotiation becomes vital for the survival of the therapy. Whether attacks are subtle or overt, it is the safety of the therapy – as potentially benign in its motives – that is at stake. Unpleasantness or fear or hate pervade; the opportunity in this is its palpable presence. Its accessibility is both a gift (it can be commented on) and a curse (it constantly threatens violence and therefore restricts freedom). Language might be used as a means to obscure or distort previously agreed-upon reflections, and to hold the therapist accountable for everything while innocence is claimed.

The potential turbulence of these therapies obscures the work to be done, presenting in its place a series of crises severed from meaning. Their aim is violent feeling rather than creativity or connection. Paradoxically, while these states may seem powerfully alive and enlivening, they in fact foreshadow deadness, the anaesthesia of the time after the storm, the toppled over houses in the wake of a hurricane. They devastate, eviscerate, regroup and begin again.

The issue here is how this kind of ruthless violence differs from the sort of destruction Winnicott suggests is essential to object usage. Certainly, if the therapist survives the storm and steadies herself for the next one, there will be a gain, but only insofar as the patient is able to take in destructiveness as the occasion for mourning, reparation and gratitude. Some, faced with devastation, are able only to reach for aliveness by placing the source of the storm outside of themselves, and therefore beyond repair. Moreover, as Bollas (1996) has described, for some patients there is an attachment made to the storm itself, so that resting states feel frighteningly numb and empty.

Becoming orange peel: the therapist's ruth and survival of ruthlessness

In "Hate in the Countertransference," Winnicott describes the baby's eager engagement with the mother as "cupboard love, so that having got what he wants he throws her away like orange peel" (Winnicott, 2002, p. 197). Survival of being used in this way requires a ruthlessness of its own. In "The Aims of Psycho-Analytical Treatment," he says, "Having begun an analysis I expect to continue with it, to survive it, and to end it" (Winnicott, 1965, p. 166). In this paper and in "Metapsychological and Clinical Aspects of Regression within the Psycho-Analytical Set-Up," Winnicott places the ruthlessness of the therapist within features of the setting; analysis is neither mothering nor friendship, and there is "hate in the strict start and finish and in the matter of fees" (Winnicott, 2002, p. 285). The therapist must also be ruthless in making herself available for the work of being preoccupied with the patient, experiencing a full range of feeling with respect to the work, reflecting on them, and not retaliating, even if provoked. The therapist's survival must be taken for granted. In other words, while the patient needs to move fluidly between object relating and object usage in the course of the treatment, the therapist must be available to become a part of the patient's blooming buzzing confusion, and yet retain her own sturdy routes to externality.

Being a therapist is an expression of ruth, repairing, and "in a constructive way" dealing with guilt (Winnicott, 2002, p. 196). In writing about the ruthlessness of object relating, before concern is established, Winnicott emphasized the carrying over of the infant through destruction into survival as part of the development of object usage. Throughout his writing, however, and in the place he gives to regression as part of the analytic process, he writes in fluidity, the movement between states of ruth and ruthlessness. Less of a focus, but equally significant, are the ways in which the therapist must also move between states of object relating, essential to receiving the patient's unconscious communications, and object usage. Object relating allows dreaming together, reverie or enactment, and is the stuff of the transference. Hate in the countertransference is an object-relating matter. Object usage is involved in the ruthlessness of maintaining the setting's boundaries, and is inherent in the externality of the analytic third, mentalizing through the storm.

There is ruthlessness in the therapist's interpretations, knowing that when they are accurate, and unseat a defence, pain will follow. Bringing early emotional states alive, and unfreezing "the failure situation" (Winnicott, 2002, p. 281), always implies pain, although there is also satisfaction in understanding and being understood.

There are a number of ways in which the mixture of ruthlessness and ruth in the therapist might become perverted. The extremes of this are relaxing the rules of the setting, on the one hand, and through guilt or pity making extraordinary accommodation, or enforcing rules without compassion, on the other. Sadism might be found in coldly delivered or premature interpretations, schizoid withdrawal into an inaccessible professional persona, or simply fright at being ruthlessly needed. Winnicott refers to this when describing analysts' reactions when faced with patients' regression: "Some crudely say: Now sit up! Pull your socks up! Come round! Talk! "Some say: unanalysable, and throw up the sponge. A mental hospital takes over" (Winnicott, 2002, p. 291). Masochism is suggested by the therapist's failure in self-care, and her enslavement to the patient's demand for care, so that she becomes orange peel, empty of nourishment to put into the work.

Using ruth and ruthlessness in thinking diagnostically

I will be arguing through the following chapters that careful reflection on the fate of ruthlessness is a useful diagnostic and predictive clinical tool. In this, I am following Winnicott's own suggestions about ways in which patients might be grouped, especially with respect to the capacity to use psychotherapy or psychoanalysis fruitfully and fully. It is not a substitute for Winnicott's classification, but an amplification of one of its aspects.

There are two assumptions central to the argument I have made. First, it assumes that in ordinary mental functioning, object relating and object usage both feature, and the fluid movement between them mediates the presence of true-self aliveness in negotiation with externality. Second, object relating (implying projection and introjection) carries channels of communication (light, air, oxygen) to a true self, which is of necessity sequestered from both the day-to-day routines of social interaction as well as the glare of consciousness. I am interpreting Winnicott here as placing the true self, and the origins of the spontaneous gesture, as operating largely as an unconscious and non-compliant originary source of aliveness. Just as object relating and object usage are always in operation, so too is the ruthlessness that is initially a feature of object relating, and responsive to true-self needs. Ruthlessness is responsible for setting in motion cycles of destruction, survival and repair that continue lifelong, and this is necessary to the creation of externality.

From this, several issues that affect patients' use of the analytic or psychotherapeutic space emerge. When there is object relating unmediated on the whole by object usage (because the stage of concern has never been reached), survival of the object and creation of externality are both in question. This has consequences for maintaining the therapeutic frame, which is firmly rooted in belief that the patient is able to move between object relating within the session and object usage in adhering to the limits of both the time offered, and ways in which the space might be used.

The quality of ruthlessness characteristic of patients in whom object usage is unstable may be used defensively as a way of walling off re-experiencing trauma. Paradoxically, this might then be the mechanism that underlies repetition of trauma, as it both signifies (points to) the area of vulnerability at the same time as it attempts to prevent its being seen and attended to. I am suggesting here that defensive ruthlessness might fruitfully be used as a way of thinking about enactment (in terms of relational theory) or transference (in terms of object relations theory).

Insofar as object usage is a developmental achievement, helping patients to reach it implies a reworking of a part of development; this suggests regression and provision of a new experience so that the patient can be carried over destruction to survival and reparation, with appropriate mourning for what has been lost. The arduousness of this, and its implications for what the therapeutic dyad will need to bear in terms of suffering, will depend on the extent of the original failure, and the form taken by the ruthlessness with which it is walled in or walled out.

Perversions of ruth also need to be considered. They involve its ruthless deployment in obscuring or subverting self-care, spontaneity and negotiation by subjugation out of pity; pitiless self-sacrifice then becomes coercive in its effects on the system.

In thinking about variations of ruthlessness in patients, it is also useful to hold in mind the ways in which the analytic situation – its setting, rules, modes of engagement and expressions of compassion – also move constantly between a pushing forward, against, through defence, and concern for the tender holding together of bits and pieces that surface. While this is always a balancing act, and will vary depending on an individual therapist's style and theory, it might from time to time become unbalanced, through the therapist's own defensive deployment of ruthlessness or collapse into ruth.

I am aware of the difficulties inherent in an approach that, with its emphasis on infancy, pushes into the background the complexities and formative effects of later life experience. It offers a potentially anthropomorphized view of the baby's experience transposed upon that of adult patient. Moreover, any form of categorization or diagnosis works against holding theory lightly, as Orange (2015) correctly enjoins us to do. Thinking about ruthlessness, however, has the capacity to add to psychoanalytic theory and technique in the following ways. It expands the ways in which we think about patients' capacity to express strong affect – always a ruthless act – and therefore to assist them in this act of communication. Just as importantly, ruthlessness is deeply implicated in the experience of autonomy, and therefore being able to experience being accountable to an emotional life. Ruthlessness is not an affect, but an action. It is entwined with the expression of love and hate, guilt and shame, rage and envy, and deserves close attention as the gathering together, expression and potential resolution of all these powerful affective events.

Note

1 Throughout Winnicott's work, he refers to "mother" as the initial caregiver. The gender and class assumptions embedded in this terminology can be undone partly by substituting the word "caregiver" when not quoting Winnicott directly. It is, however, critical that in writing about mother/baby units in the first months of life, Winnicott's argument assumes a single caregiver "preoccupied" with the baby as a primary task, and this is not easily translated into situations in which multiple caregivers for babies are economically a necessity. Moreover, the terms resonate semantically in ways that do not always fit well with the affective field Winnicott so vividly describes. For this chapter, I have therefore made the decision to keep the word "mother" throughout, and to note that it is problematic. Wherever I can in other chapters, I use the word "caregiver."

References

Allen, J. G., Fonagy, P. and Bateman, A. W. (2008). *Mentalizing in clinical practice.* American Psychiatric Publications.

Benjamin, J. (2017). *Beyond doer and done to: Recognition theory, intersubjectivity and the third.* Routledge.

Bollas, C. (1996). Borderline desire. *International Forum of Psychoanalysis*, *5*(1), 5–10.

Bromberg, P. M. (2013). *Awakening the dreamer: Clinical journeys*. Routledge.

Eigen, M. (1981). The area of faith in Winnicott, Lacan and Bion. *The International Journal of Psycho-Analysis*, *62*(4), 413–433.

Eigen, M. (2001). *Damaged bonds*. Karnac.

Eigen, M. (2004). *Psychic deadness*. Karnac.

Fonagy, P. (2000). Attachment and borderline personality disorder. *Journal of the American PsychoanalyticPassociation*, *48*(4), 1129–1146.

Fonagy, P. (2006). The mentalization-focused approach to social development. In J. G. Allen and P. Fonagy (Eds.), *The handbook of mentalization-based treatment* (pp. 53–100). John Wiley & Sons.

Fonagy, P. and Campbell, C. (2015). Bad blood revisited: Attachment and psychoanalysis. *British Journal of Psychotherapy*, *31*(2), 229–250.

Ghent, E. (1990). Masochism, submission, surrender: Masochism as a perversion of surrender. *Contemporary Psychoanalysis*, *26*(1), 108–136.

James, W. (2013). *The principles of psychology*. Read Books.

Joseph, B. (1989). *Psychic equilibrium and psychic change: Selected papers of Betty Joseph* (Vol. *9*). Psychology Press.

Kohut, H. (1971). *The analysis of the self: A systematic approach to the psychoanalytic treatment of narcissistic personality disorders*. University of Chicago Press.

Lachmann, F. M. and Beebe, B. (2013). Representational and selfobject transferences: A developmental perspective. In A. Goldberg (Ed.), *Progress in self psychology, Vol. 8: New therapeutic visions* (pp. 3–15). Analytic Press.

Lucente, R. L. (1998). A Winnicottian approach to intimacy in the therapeutic alliance. *Journal of Analytic Social Work*, *5*(2), 19–33.

Mitchell, S. A. (2014). *Relationality: From attachment to intersubjectivity*. Routledge.

Ogden, T. H. (1997). Reverie and interpretation. *Psychoanalytic Quarterly, 66*(4), 567–595.
Ogden, T. H. (2012). *Creative readings: Essays on seminal analytic works*. Routledge.
Ogden, T. H. (2014). *Rediscovering psychoanalysis: Thinking and dreaming, learning and forgetting*. Routledge.
Ogden, T. H. (2016). *Reclaiming unlived life: Experiences in psychoanalysis*. Routledge.
Orange, D. M. (2011). *The suffering stranger: Hermeneutics for everyday clinical practice*. Routledge.
Orange, D. M. (2015). *Nourishing the inner life of clinicians and humanitarians: The ethical turn in psychoanalysis*. Routledge.
Pizer, S. A. (2013). *Building bridges: The negotiation of paradox in psychoanalysis*. Routledge.
Racker, H. (2012). *Transference and countertransference*. Karnac.
Slochower, J. (2013). *Holding and psychoanalysis: A relational perspective*. Routledge.
Stern, D. B. (2013). *Unformulated experience: From dissociation to imagination in psychoanalysis* (Vol. *8*). Routledge.
Wallin, D. J. (2007). *Attachment in psychotherapy*. Guilford Press.
Winnicott, D. W. (1965). *The maturational processes and the facilitating environment: Studies in the theory of emotional development*. Karnac.
Winnicott, D. W. (1969). The use of an object. *The International Journal of Psycho-Analysis, 50*, 711–716.
Winnicott, D. W. (1971). *Playing and reality*. Psychology Press.
Winnicott, D. W. (1989). *Psycho-analytic explorations*, ed. C. Winnicott, R. Shepherd and M. Davis. Karnac.
Winnicott, D. W. (1990). *Home is where we start from: Essays by a psychoanalyst*. WW Norton & Company.
Winnicott, D. W. (2002). *Through paediatrics to psychoanalysis: Collected papers*. Karnac.

Chapter 2

Ruthlessness and idealization

This chapter takes forward several ideas about the ways in which psychoanalytic psychotherapy might carry a patient over from the magical but nutrient-empty space of "magical introjection" to being in the therapeutic space for the purpose of achieving "use" in its fullest sense, destroying through this use, surviving, and finally creating meaning with the "immense joy" of which Winnicott speaks (Winnicott, 1969, p. 711). It begins by elaborating on forms of ruthless idealization that prevent the therapeutic space from being used as a space that will survive the vagaries of rupture and multiplicity. It considers the kinds of interventions during this stage of the work that may set the platform for the shift from object relating to object usage. This includes discussing the fate of interpretation with idealizing patients. It ends with some comments about the cost of de-idealization, especially with respect to psychic deadness. To argue the case, I will introduce case material from two treatments, each of which had idealization in the treatment as a core feature.

Idealization as a ruthless defence against taking in and being taken in

Idealization has many purposes, and is an ordinary part of human interaction (Slochower, 2011). It serves primary maternal preoccupation by infusing mothers with love for an infant, uncluttered by doubt about upheaval and the indignities of interruption. It shelters preschoolers encountering the lives of families not their own by convincing them that their parents are the richest, smartest and most beautiful in the land. It launches us into adult love affairs, untroubled by niggling irritations in moments of misunderstanding and during conversational glitches. It allows us to follow leaders into adventures and elections, trusting their capacity to guide and guard. It gives essential fuel to protest movements working towards passionately held goals. Most of all, it protects each one of us from our own deep fallibilities in facing a precarious and unknowable future. In short, benign idealization is the tender vessel through which optimism is sustained.

Primary optimism, this buffer against the overwhelming emotion of early life, underlies possibilities of thriving, and has a long history in psychoanalytic theory. For Freud, it mediates the flow of libido between object and ego, and functionally sets up ideals through identifications. It is a process essential both to the setting up of the superego, and more broadly the regulation of self-esteem (Freud, 1914; Spruiell, 1979, p. 789). For Klein, in her own words, "idealization is an essential process in the young child's mind, since he cannot yet cope in any other way with his fears of persecution (a result of his own hatred)" (Klein, 1940, p. 130). This line of thinking is elaborated in Kernberg's approach to idealization as a so-called "primitive" defence against a world infused with danger, and as protection against both rage and envy (Kernberg, 1974).[1] Idealization of objects protects against fantasies of being attacked; simultaneously, the formation of a grandiose self that denies dependence serves as a protection against the ravaging effects of envy (Mitchell, 1986, p. 109).

The other line of theoretical development is built around the idea of defence against injury rather than aggression. In this genealogy, idealization is a defence against frailty, especially during periods of dependence. For Kohut, idealization is an essential part of a developmental environment in which the self needs access to a self-object imbued with the capacity to soothe. Such idealization gives way gradually to a more reality-based relationship, so long as failures are not too traumatic. Moreover, it leads to the firm establishment of ideals as an ordinary part of healthy adult life. This view echoes Freud's early formulations of idealization as a route to the formation of ego-ideals (Kohut, 1971). Acceptance of patients' need to idealize their analyst, and to place optimism in the outcome of their treatment squarely in a trusted and soothing setting, re-establishes an interrupted and necessary developmental trajectory. A Kohutian view of idealization slants us towards the realm of hope in engaging with inevitably painful therapeutic exploration, and takes the edge off dread.

The 1970s debate between Kohut and Kernberg, and their elaboration in subsequent decades about origins and treatment of narcissistic patients, and technical aspects of managing idealization in treatments, can usefully be divided into theory that deals with the origins and treatment of narcissistic disorders or disorders of the self, and that which focuses specifically on idealization as a defence.

The relational tradition has embraced both poles of this debate, emphasizing both the importance of providing a holding environment that encourages the needed new relationship and also the exploration of the full range of experience that underpins repetition of relational dilemmas (Slochower, 2011; Stern, 1994). This entails the capacity of treatments to hold idealization as a potential well of creative (if illusory) energy, and to be responsive to the invitation to unfold the array of feelings, both positive and negative, lying behind it. In Mitchell's view, the therapeutic task involves integration of both idealization and grandiosity into ordinary self-esteem, as well as searching for the reasons for the original defensive fractures (Mitchell, 1986):

> The most useful response entails a subtle dialectic between joining the patient in the narcissistic integration and also simultaneously questioning the nature and purpose of that integration, both a playful participation in the patient's illusions and a puzzled curiosity about how and why they came to be the *sine qua non* of the analysand's sense of security and involvements with others.
>
> (Mitchell, 1986, p. 125)

It is worth stressing here that idealization deployed in the service of facilitating buoyancy in negotiation of challenge may well allow relational engagement, whereas idealization warding off early agonies is altogether less permeable, and in fact prevents relational negotiation altogether. This differentiation makes a significant difference to the technical challenges and experience of the transference in idealizing patients (Gedo, 1975; Slochower, 2011).

In this landscape, Winnicott seems to be a seamless predecessor to Kohut, although he seldom referred to idealization explicitly. It is nonetheless deeply implicated in his views of development, and is best captured in his description of the "good breast" experiences. In "Metapsychological and Clinical Aspects of Regression within the Psycho-Analytical Set-Up," he describes how these "help the child to tide over short periods in which the mother fails" (Winnicott, 2002, p. 276). The child's access to ruthless use of the breast depends in the first instance of her capacity to hallucinate it when it is needed, and this is itself an omnipotent transformation of a world designed to assuage on demand. Gradual disillusionment (or in other words, de-idealization of the mother's capacity to anticipate and meet every need as it is felt) comes only when the infant/child is able to sustain him or herself inwardly with internalized resources. In "Notes Made on the Train, Part 2," Winnicott suggests that attempts to preserve the object, rather than using it with the "guilt relative to the destructive ideas that go with loving," is idealization. It has its counterpart in "a rendering down of the object from perfection towards badness," a denigration that paradoxically preserves a state of object relating (Winnicott, 1989, p. 231).

Regardless of how theorists place idealization as part of ordinary development and human relatedness, there is general agreement that it becomes a focus for intervention when it introduces significant distortion into relational engagement. In Winnicottian terms, when magical thinking or hallucination predominate, object usage is impossible, and the self cannot be replenished through relational exchange. This also implies difficulty with use of potential space, with all the freedoms this confers. Excessive dependence on an idealizing defence might take the form of an inability to experience or express anger, depletion of self at the expense of the idealized other, excessive self-sacrifice and withering of ambition, a striving to live up to an internalized ideal with consequent perfectionism that hampers creativity and spontaneity, or inability to sustain intimate connection with its necessary messiness and ambivalence. It always implies the shadowy presence, managed through projection, of a haughty and omnipotent self that is sequestered but denigrates the world it looks out upon (Akhtar, 1996; Bromberg, 1983; Kernberg, 1974; Kohut, 1971; Mitchell, 1986). This vital link between idealization and grandiosity, operating in a dynamic relation with one another, is made explicit in Kohutian theory, but is evident, implicitly or explicitly, in all the theories I have referred to above.

The link with ruthlessness lies in the controlling effects of idealization. All the more seductive for its rosiness, it nonetheless pinions the person so conceived into a particular "narrative rigidity" that brooks no counter-narrative, no hint of ambivalence or disappointment (Stern, 2010, p. 13). The therapist becomes incorporated into this rigidity. The content of an exchange will automatically be received as wise and good, although its links with changes to affective colouring or behavioural change over time will be missing. As Bach points out, analysts working with narcissistic patients relying on grandiose self-presentation or idealization "sometimes develop an intense feeling of frustration about the impermanence of even their effective interpretations and compare it with talking into the wind or writing on the sand, only to have one's words effaced moments later by the waves" (Bach, 1977, p. 209). As Akhtar (1996) describes in his paper on work with "someday" and "if only" fantasies, the idealization might take the form of nostalgia about a perfect past kept alive in the patient's mind as paradise lost, and relived as a way of avoiding engagement with an imperfect present, or longing for *deus ex machina* solutions to current problems. The therapist's attempts to dismantle these fantasies prematurely will be either ignored altogether or experienced as a form of attack.

There is one additional rigidity inserted into the idealizing narrative, and this is central to its coercive quality. To present oneself as enslaved to the wisdom of a therapist leaves no room for negotiation or flexibility of meanings; this in turn opens the way for sadomasochistic displays of bewilderment when suggestions miss the mark, or interpretations, used as instructions, cause mishaps and collisions in relating or living. So, for example, a patient and therapist discuss together the patient's experience of being neglected emotionally by her parents when a child. She then confronts her aged parents with this "insight" from her therapy, tagging the therapist's exploration as opinion or judgement, rather than the shifting fact/fiction of a psychoanalytic discussion. Chaos ensues, the patient here being a "violent innocent," stirring strong feeling and stepping away from its effects. The whole scene is then reported back to the therapist, and the circle is complete, with idealization and a taunting denigration intricately layered (Bollas, 2013).

I turn now to two clinical examples, and then to a consideration of the ways in which thinking about ruthlessness might be of benefit in working with the idealizing patient.

The activist

This patient was an activist, and a multiskilled, tireless worker on community projects, many headed by colleagues and friends. Without wealth and intensely private, but sometimes in the public eye, she guarded her solitude and her highly principled way of life, which demanded a strict monitoring of all she participated in. She supported a talented generation of idealists, many needing a project to fulfil a brimming sense of purpose. She had skill in giving those she worked with the sense that she had merely fostered their own ideas, and given to them a context in which they could grow. She was not dissembling in this: her idealizing belief in those with whom she was involved did allow creativity to flourish. She had difficulty, however, in measuring the contribution of her own gifts of insight and skill to the emerging products.

She promised all who consulted with her the kind of meaning that is invested specifically in the creation of new things: new landscapes, new hope, and a willingness to take on inertia, corruption or self-promotion. Apart from attending to the management of projects being dreamed into being, and quickening the life in them, she carried with her such belief in her powers that she had come to be worshipped as the source of success itself. She was visited by men and women from far and wide, and at times she complained that she was depleted, and that her capacity to organize and inspire was wearing thin.

Of course, I received this account from her, and noticed that it had the frills and frolics of a rosy picture; in short, it was not free from puffery. Nonetheless, such was my activist's fame that word of her skill reached me through acquaintances.

In her creation of lives for others, there were two paths. For some, she supported and attended, and the birth of a successful project was then celebrated. For others, her task was more difficult: she needed to actually find a viable project, insist on its viability, and place it in the hands of the person in search of a cause, a place to invest energy. Far more than attending as a helper, she was part-mother, part-visionary, conjuring groups and movement forward from small seeds. Somehow, she convinced all her colleagues that this was not her work, but theirs, merely a channelling, generously bequeathed. She asked for little in return but the fees she needed to travel to the next project.

There was magic in the whole scene – its crises and labour, its tears and drama and public acclaim. As she left each scene, she made sure her footprints were erased as she withdrew. In her performance of every project's drama for my benefit, there was also a kind of narrative closure and a tying up of ends. She seemed genuinely triumphant about the successes of projects that sailed into the world as the work of others, and happy to bask in reflected glory. At times, there were glimmers of envy, angry asides about ways in which she had not been fully acknowledged as essential to a project's success. Sometimes she claimed ruefully that envious attacks on her during childhood by troubled cousins had cured her of any wish to be a publicly visible figure. This was the nub of the problem. We could not forever live in this enthralling and dramatic activist world, suffused with happy endings, which she simultaneously owned and disowned as her own doing. There was suffering to be had.

She had come to me with suffering: no matter what she tried, she was unable to bring to life little projects that were entirely her own. They began and faltered. Where she had some success, it was in curating and collating the work of the many she had inspired. She seldom articulated her need to head a project dreamed of, organized and brought to fruition entirely through her own efforts. She kept herself so immersed in the work of others that there seemed no time for her own ambition.

The scene was defensively ruthless in its coercion. I was in thrall to both the spectacle and the emerging need for her to find her own originality, entertained, then worried by turns. The creative and fertile in others, the abject and stunted, were all of a piece, locked into each other, light and shadow. She dazzled and distracted attention from her own ungainly failure to create for herself by intervention in the affairs of others. This is as Winnicott describes in "The Child in Health and Crisis" (Winnicott, 1965, p. 71).

She seldom gave me a role in either arena. I had some experience in the activist world, and was convinced of the considerable skill she brought to the work she was doing. In this sense, I was a credible witness for her; there were times when she made it clear that she assumed we shared a common activist agenda, and this allowed her to trust me. When I commented on the many ways in which she disowned her accomplishments and deferred work on projects of her own, she would point out the urgency of the activist work, and its significance politically. She refused to entertain for long the anxiety of making space for her own work to grow in depth and scope. As sessions with her unfolded, she seldom required comment: she filled every moment with her crisis-filled and busy life. There were times when I felt as irrelevant as orange peel, as Winnicott describes in "Hate in the Countertransference" (Winnicott, 2002, p. 201). The idealization coating her roles in her world of important causes, and her idealization of her protégées and projects, and the narrative closure of her accounts, left little for me to do except sit idly by. At the same time, I occasionally would see in her face a sense of dread when I looked as if I might speak. From this, I knew that she filled the room with stories in order to prevent an imagined blow from falling.

In two respects, she cobbled me into the sun and the moon of her life. She diligently attended her sessions, and often asked for extra times when in a crisis, so I was sure that my role as witness was significant to her. Second, she took up whatever I said, and held on to it in an idealized way. In fact, she repeated it until it lost all meaning – a passing truth turned into a truism. In those times, I was more than orange peel – I became the ears of the velveteen rabbit of the children's story, worn thin with rubbing. I might say, for example, "While on the beach, did you have a swim?" This would come back to me over and over as a spell that I cast on her behalf. "Remember you told me to swim? I have been swimming every day!" She reported that she told her friends, "My therapist says I must swim." And indeed, the swimming seemed to be helpful for a period of time. Her obedience was a taunt, a prescription dubiously followed, and my alarm at being cast as a pharmacist of spells hastened my retreat into caution.

One could think of this as the therapy space being used as potential space, my words the transitional object that carries the baby over from dependence to separation, merging and hallucinating the breast into an external world with real soft velveteen ears to be rubbed. This was partly accurate, except that in this case I had no confidence that I was being used in a transitional way, forestalling terror in the temporary absence of a good enough pair of arms. Certainly, I was being reassured of my usefulness as a rabbit. There were many times when I thought that what I was seeing was a wild creature, fobbed off with a piece of terry cloth. Was there an original experience of being mothered? And given the barriers of idealization between us, how could I carry her back into dependence and holding, and forward into taking me in, not as a truism, but as something true?

In this situation, what is the role of an interpretation? At first, it seemed there was no role at all. My words about her mind seemed baffling to her and were quickly discarded. Instructions, on the other hand, fabricated often from suggestions or questions, were put to use ruthlessly and taunted me with the precarity of the ground.

The stockbroker

Another example of idealization and its effects is illustrated by the case of a man in the cowboy world of trade. He grew up with a family trading in local markets, driving trucks of supplies to town squares, but segregated by apartheid policies from living or working in middle-class white suburbs. There were good times, however, and wealth accrued. Gradually, in the family, overalls changed into suits, and trade became all paper. Deals were made through conversations over cappuccino, a veneer of brotherhood veiling threats and burying virtual assassinations. Many lawyers were hired to deal with tax and debt and occasional bits and pieces that went the way of bankruptcy and lawsuits.

It was a world replete with both rules, honourable and dishonourable, and rule-breaking, one leading inevitably to the other as money changed hands over and over. The rules and transparency of trading on the exchange had a dark web of networks and sleights of hand, imaginary ceilings being broken through, and rumours inflating this stock and deflating that. To guide him, my patient had an army of consultants – highly paid stock market experts and strategists and academic economists and politicians who urged brothers in business into smarter, slicker and more risky performances. I was told therefore of a suited, ruthless and at times unethical world. It was a competitive world, and he was a sporting man; my head filled with sporting metaphors every time we met.

The sayings of experts, sounding oddly folksy given their hard-nosed credentials, spread over the conversation like almond oil: "Emotionally, I need to push my comfort zone in this project," he would say. "He's given me the opportunity of seeing my inner bear." "I want to inspire, not manage, my people." "He's my accountability buddy; I'll check in with him about what you're saying on this one."

Occasionally, aggression erupted beyond the furious drive forward that is encased in the language of the deal. My patient described a moment when a would-be client barged into him as he walked down a corridor towards his office, smiled, and apologized as if it had been an accident. My patient was sure it was deliberate and reacted savagely, as if he had been punched. He grabbed the man by his suit lapels and shook him. He was like a terrier with a rat clamped in his jaws. He shouted, "Don't you *ever f*****g* do that again!" This was an explosion of which he was proud, and he assumed my approbation, without waiting to see if it would come.

Quieter shows of violence pleased him too. He said to one of his younger staff members:

> I want to be clear here, this is my business, and I will run it as I wish. When I want your input, I will ask you for it. Now you will leave this meeting without saying one more word.

As with the activist, who owned and disowned her considerable strengths, he lived in a split world. He had a stellar career, at least according to his own account. He was wealthy, drove expensive cars, and lived in a mansion next to the sea. He had rages, barely managing to keep himself from hitting men in his path, but he felt this was expected in his trade world and served his business. In other words, he presented himself as a colossus. But then there was the slippery slide of his dependence on the approbation of men he idealized, all the ways in which he got affirmations from buddies, talk lathered with languages of business-mindfulness, a world in which he made idols of consultants and royalty of politicians.

He worked constantly on a set of internal landscapes, polishing their mirrors, a world growing more and more elaborate and cluttered with words for feelings and reflections on reflections, goals and colour charts of steps to success and personality types, and top 10 indicators of high-stakes surfing. Everything in this landscape was presented as rational. He smiled knowingly when I suggested that even on the stock exchange, the irrational and chaotic has a place. He allowed me these quaint notions as my special toy to play with.

There was another side to his split world. He sometimes felt uncomfortable for a moment or two, as he was oddly demeaned in his marriage. His wife had no truck with second-guessing stock market trends; neither did she care about how much money he made. He was sidelined in the working of the house and told to speak quietly so that he did not wake the sleeping children. Although he referred constantly to his marital happiness, it was clear that he had suffered a demotion at home, and this was a thorn in the lion's paw.[2]

In the therapy, he prompted me to act as yet another organizational expert or strategist, to provide him with another layer of mentorship. There was ruthlessness both in the positioning and also in the idealization of a particular way of thinking. This was achieved through ritual design crafted carefully, a careful order of speaking that rehearsed the session before and envisioned the one ahead. From time to time, I was rewarded with compliments about my wisdom. At the end of the time, he gave me a summary of what he had heard. Idealization of the rules of psychoanalytic psychotherapy and the insights he assured me I offered him was set against the production of a series of formulae for success, reproduced from a variety of bestselling books. My words were filtered through a narrative thick with apparent mindfulness but turned into junk status unless they matched exactly one of the guru-sentences for which his appetite seemed endless. And while he reported on the inflammation of his paw, he quickly turned this too into a sequence of problem-solving steps.

Interpretations seemed to penetrate only as the clichés they were quickly turned into. Occasionally, if I spoke gravely, and preached like a guru, I suspected a word or two slipped through.

Matters of technique

> "Real isn't how you are made," said the Skin Horse. "It's a thing that happens to you. When a child loves you for a long, long time, not just to play with, but REALLY loves you, then you become Real."
>
> "Does it hurt?" asked the Rabbit.
>
> "Sometimes," said the Skin Horse, for he was always truthful. "When you are Real you don't mind being hurt."
>
> "Does it happen all at once, like being wound up," he asked, "or bit by bit?"
>
> "It doesn't happen all at once," said the Skin Horse. "You become. It takes a long time. That's why it doesn't happen often to people who break easily, or have sharp edges, or who have to be carefully kept. Generally, by the time you are Real, most of your hair has been loved off, and your eyes drop out and you get loose in the joints and very shabby. But these things don't matter at all, because once you are Real you can't be ugly, except to people who don't understand."
>
> (Williams, 1922, p. 3)

There are a number of considerations to be taken into account when thinking about ruth and ruthlessness in the treatment of patients for whom idealization is a significant defence. First of all, for almost all patients, idealization is a benign backdrop to initial parts of engaging in the therapy, trusting the setting, the therapist's expertise, adherence to professional codes of conduct, and capacity to understand. This constitutes the holding environment and is an essential foundation to building a potential space within which to create. Moreover, idealization might feature from time to time, and in ways that "tide over" the patient at times of crisis, or during patches of very painful exploration. These are quite distinct from the relentlessness of an idealization that incorporates everything that the therapist has to say as "sayings," awesome truths that become truisms, comments adored and then aligned to a fictionalized narrative, or simply "a jumble of words" (Bach, 1977, p. 209). In this way, the idealized contributions of the therapist are fitted to content already known, or, in Winnicott's terms, become as if hallucinated by the patient, because the match between what is said, heard and internalized seals further an already sealed system. In short, there is no new news, no insight that penetrates the patient's defences or continuity of being, and yet there is also an addictive attachment to the incorporation of words as things.

This ruthless laundering of the therapist's words into that which is perfection might be experienced as "new" insight, but is merely confirmatory of what has always been known. It has a parallel in the grandiose patient's use of the space. In Kernberg's description:

> The narcissistic patient extends his own grandiosity to include the analyst, and thus, while apparently free associating in the presence of the analyst, really talks to himself expanded into a grandiose "self-observing" figure to which the patient becomes, temporarily, an attachment or satellite.
>
> (Kernberg, 1974, p. 221)

A Kernbergian approach suggests early confrontation with both positive and negative aspects of the transference, including the patient's need to keep the analyst at a distance through idealization, and systematically interpreting destructive impulses, specifically envy and rage. Survival of its expression, and confrontation with the patchy satisfactions of the real world, is key to Kernberg's approach. He argues:

> [The] prominent reason why these patients cannot tolerate facing their feelings of hatred and envy is because they think such feelings would destroy the analyst, destroy their hope for a good relationship with him, and crush their hope of being helped.
>
> (Kernberg, 1974, p. 262)

Kernberg's approach is technically ruthless, although it implies an understanding of the patient's dilemma that is replete with ruthful compassion.

While Kernberg's approach suggests this as a productive path, others are advocates of a slower building of internal resources, after which the defences will become more flexible of their own accord (Kohut, 1971; Slochower, 2013).

The process of idealization brings with it a constant reminder of the patient's need to hallucinate a feed, and at the same time the fact of no food being exchanged. There is an addictive quality to the routine of insight being fobbed off as magic in an endless cycle. At the same time, there is a rumbling threat that catastrophic disruption of the defence with premature interpretation might catapult the patient into material that cannot be experienced without destabilizing anxiety.

The paradox of threatening fragility lies in the robust effectiveness of the idealizing defence. Interpretations, except perhaps those that directly confront the patient with their envy and rage, often seem to have no impact at all, except as fuel to the guru-making machinery. As Bromberg suggests, penetrating an idealizing defence, or its twin, a grandiose self-presentation, is "an inch by inch process" (Bromberg, 1983, p. 378). Bromberg suggests that poorly timed interventions in the narrative rigidities of patients and analysts caught between mirroring grandiosity or clinging on to idealizations are:

> indistinguishable from an attempt by the "all-knowing" parent to disqualify their reality and leave them with nothing but whatever selfishness and failure is being attributed to their behaviour at that moment. These are individuals for whom the content of an interpretation directed towards a resistance will be processed as a sign of the analyst's narcissism; an instance of non-responsiveness to them, and a failure to appreciate or value them simply for who they are.
>
> (Bromberg, 1983, p. 378)

Both the fragility and the impenetrability of the defensive idealization have to be kept in mind: linked dynamically, they change both over the course of the therapy, and in response to events in the patient's life. This is an "empathy/anxiety" gradient to be managed.

Akhtar offers technique designed to dismantle "someday" and "as if" fantasies defensive against narcissistic disequilibrium. It combines provision of an opportunity to consolidate a self threatened with disintegration, and gradual confrontation with the need to abandon idealized fantasy states. He suggests a staged approach:

> (1) providing and sustaining a meaningful "holding environment"; (2) employing "affirmative interventions"; (3) interpreting the defensive, narcissistic and masochistic aspects of idealization inherent in the two fantasies; (4) rupturing the patient's excessive hope, analyzing the effects of such rupture, and facilitating the resultant mourning; (5) reconstructing the early scenarios underlying the need for excessive hope; and (6) paying careful attention to the countertransference feelings.
>
> (Akhtar, 1996, p. 747)

In this way, the scene is set for a period of holding and swimming along with an idealizing atmosphere that coerces as it entices, with the hovering shadows of eruption or disintegration keeping the frail edifice in place, inching through affirmation and holding towards a scene in which survival cannot be taken for granted.

Inch by inch with the activist

With the activist, my task was to turn my velveteen ears into real ears, and my sentences into the stuff of play. We both needed to get hurt, and not to mind, because we were Real.

For a very long time, I held her and provided "affirmative interventions'" in the sense that I did not often challenge the fantasy of the idealized world in which she lived, one in which some day there might be fair resources for all. With occasional crises, her work fell into patterns that avoided tumult, and in small ways she was able to bring something of herself into projects she managed, by shaping them in particular ways. I was, however, still extravagantly entertained by her witchery, and enjoyed her company; this lulled me into overvaluing our small achievements and assuming these may be the only steps we could take. It may be that her apparently impenetrable idealizations of the therapy had the effect of setting in motion a regulatory counterbalance in me, as if I needed to insist on small incremental gains as being the most our work together would achieve.

From time to time, when she encountered vulnerable and adoring people in her project path, she fell in love, and the haze of romance and flutters of the heart filled the therapy with light tenderness. These times were at first so rosy and their heavy perfume so saturated the air that I had no doubt that idealizing fantasies were afoot. At some point, the romance cracked, and there was heartbreak, always unforeseen. Blame was apportioned – not to the would-be lover, who remained idealized, but to events, travel, storms, unpleasant family members. After an episode of love, there followed a profound withdrawal, first to bed, then to routines of work, and changes in setting, redecorating and gardening. A kind of pseudo-mourning took place, an embrace of ageing, solitariness and loss, a kind of elaborate wake at which she was a lively and deeply enlivening corpse who startled the mourners with her capacity to throw a heavenly party. Her periods in widow's weeds she relished as steps in a journey; I saw only a circle, only repetitions, and more losses of the same kind to come.

So lacy were these years of engagement, and yet so ruthless in their unfolding, their insistence on a single way, sips from the chalice of rosiness, that I was in danger of becoming unresponsive, and folded into a sense of futility. Time came, though, when there was a fleeting clue that something more active and forthright than a holding environment was needed. I knew this was such a moment because of a second's pause between her sentences and my background vocalizations; I saw in her face a new tension and attention, a reaching for contact. It was a moment when biography edged out fiction, and there was new news. The sliver widened – like an eclipse of a paper sun.

Fatigue about working in the service of others, and a growing impulse to work for herself, presented for a time of depressed mood. We began to explore, tentatively at first, the consequences of putting aside her being indentured to others' projects in order to explore new ventures of her own. She had many reasons why this was impossible: the many people she would let down, the improbability of her succeeding on her own. She began to explore the terrain, though, at first through quiet conversations with friends, and then more publicly, in voicing her dreams on social media platforms.

At first, it seemed that her move towards working for herself, owning her ambition, was destined to be turned into another version of previous attempts, all of which became collations and celebrations of the projects of others. She met my comments on her avoidance of envious attack by minimizing exposure of her originality with intellectual curiosity, but without changing significantly her usual busy life of servitude and activism on others' behalf. I would raise her dream for herself, but knew that my probes were in danger of becoming orders, and hence not the spontaneous gesture we sought. I was also conscious that she might idealize a version of a project she believed we had dreamed up together, and launch herself into it in a risky way, exposing herself to the possibility of failure and criticism from those in her circles.

At this time, there were sessions in which anger and mourning occasionally featured in her reports of her busy life. Her rebellion against complying with the ruthless demands of launching a project surfaced as a new firmness with deadlines and rules for payment. She mourned lost opportunities to take charge in the past, to insist that her careful crafting into order of others' jumbled plans be seen as in itself an act of originality. At this time, too, she took on occasional apprentices, ostensibly to help her with an increasingly unwieldy set of demands. She handed over to them many of the skills she had learned in her career, but she also began naming with them, and for them, a role not as merely a project manager, but its creative energy too. She fell in love with teaching them, but more importantly, with them as proxies of herself in various situations, she began to find time for creative adventures of her own.

This had immediate implications for the relationship between us in the therapy. There were times when she insisted, albeit with laughter, that I had "forbidden" her to do anything but work on her new venture. There were times, too, when she tried to draw me directly into it by asking me to listen to draft proposals or to comment on strategic plans. My attempts to be affirming of her willingness to explore new possibilities for herself were interpreted as a declaration that her work was destined to be a great success; here, she interpellated me into the "excessive hope" that Akhtar suggests needs "rupturing" (Akhtar, 1996, p. 747). She resisted any rupture by screening out my presence in the conversation about her hopes, by filling the time with reports on apparently urgent matters. During this phase, when there were disappointments in the process, she simply discarded me as a sounding board and turned to others for comfort. However, as she became more secure in managing her business, less preoccupied with the effects of her growing success on others she imagined to be envious of her, and convinced of her survival when there were temporary defeats and hurdles, she gradually became less inclined to transform all our interactions in the therapy into writs or tokens of a sanctified exchange. As idealization receded in its constraining effect, bit by bit we began to spend more time in sessions on the origins of her anxiety, and its working through in the relationship with me.

In the latter part of our work together, the activist and I had often talked about the way in which her difficulty in being ambitious and seeking success had been shaped by the destructive relationship with her cousins, one of whom in particular had envied her and attacked her achievements. The conflicts between her and her cousins were acknowledged, but her parents gave her no support as she struggled increasingly with fear of displaying any of her achievements at home. It became apparent that her ruthless retreat into imagined, idealized triumphs, on behalf of others, was a defence against the pain of a childhood in which her parents avoided celebrating her achievements; moreover, the conflict with the cousins was hard to unravel because it replicated similar difficulty in the preceding generation.

When the activist began to show more of herself at work, and to talk more directly about her family and childhood, she found it difficult to differentiate between internal battles to be fought and lived through in the therapy, and a desire to be ruthless in the world. She severed all connection with her cousins, consigning their communications to junk mail. She wrote stern emails to her parents, berating them for having failed to protect her. There was also turbulence in our relationship, as she longed for me to take her side and urge her into further confrontations. As time went by, and as she settled with a new relationship with parents slowly becoming dependent and frail, her survival without the barricade of idealization began to become a possibility.

Sparring with the stockbroker

It was like playing basketball with an agile, athletic giant. He ran his own sessions, basketing his insights with a stretch of an arm. The ball was not mine to have, although there would be no game if I was not there. To even up the odds against me, he was gracious in attributing his play to my passes; he treated me as being on his team.

The insights accumulated; they ratcheted up so swiftly that they were barely recorded, and were certainly his rather than mine. Afraid of the glowering rage that flared when he felt affronted or diminished in any way, I was very circumspect with my interventions. Occasionally, I got in the way of his sailing towards the next basket by tripping him with a thought or a question. Invariably, he regrouped quickly, telling me he anticipated that thought.

The paradox was that he presented himself in two ways. He was absolutely independent, a solo player with an extraordinary scoreline, knowing everything. Equally, he was deeply dependent on his mirroring experts, me among them, his idealized scaffolds. I was there to witness the first as I wore the attribution of expertise, even as I was prevented from doing expert work.

This was the pattern for many months until a change in his work circumstances necessitated a period of living on another continent. For a time, we lost touch altogether. When we came together again, we were somewhat new to each other. He had been sobered by his experience abroad, and although he did not say this specifically, his ambitions seemed to have new boundaries. I, too, felt readier to survive the forms of ruthlessness with which I was being asked to grapple.

Our encounters began to take a familiar shape: I was idealized but also teased and taunted in being reminded how experts thought about the world's problems. I began to use the expert status he often attributed to me as an enabler rather than a coercive restraint. I ruthlessly made use of my experience and theoretical knowledge to engage with him when he framed his talk in the words of bestselling authors. Occasionally, I hit a tender spot, and he tucked a thought away to chew over privately, telling me loftily he would reflect on it and come back to me. I was imperiously treated after these conversations.

Then there was a catastrophe: he lost status in his stock-trading world and felt betrayed by his experts and mentors. There was trouble at home too: his wife demanded a more nuanced and sensitive presence from him as father of her children, something less entitled and more empathic. He retreated from the therapy for some months, claiming travel and a full schedule as problems in getting to see me. When he eventually returned, I found he listened more and was a solemn presence. My feelings now fell into two pieces. There was dread of his rage, which permeated my thoughts before each session. I imagined him towering over me, red-faced and shouting. The other piece in me was both fond and firm. As I began to believe in myself, and signalled a new resilience, we began the work of making links between the flares of rage he reported (and I dreaded) and a childhood of strict rules that precluded tenderness. The idealized fabric of his childhood narrative gave way to "spots of commonness" (Eliot, 1961), parents driven by ambition rather than idealism, with scant time for a child's frights and fear. As he began to unearth memories of a family deeply affected by racist policies in apartheid's segregationist past, and his family's determination to give him an excellent education, he began to recall his joy and fear about the neighbourhood in which he had grown up, his awareness of its texture as an embattled community, and also the vigilance required by his family and friends to protect their home against intrusion. As we reached this point, I heard less often about experts and consultants, and more about his own need for affirmation as he rebuilt his business. He allowed me to reframe "someday" fantasies, in which he would be an influential player on the stock exchanges of the world, in terms of everyday deals, with losses as part of the expected course of global markets. His survival into this new space of play brought with it curiosity about and tolerance of his children's experimentation with defiance and demand; in surviving their ruthlessness, his own sense of ruth began to be a resource for him both at work and at home.

Truth breaking in: the sad consequences of being real

In Eliot's *Middlemarch*, the novel Virginia Woolf described as "one of the few English novels written for grown-up people" (Woolf, 2017), Dorothea Brooke, an extraordinary study in idealism and idealization, has the passion and intelligent will to reflect on her own failings. After a night of such reflection, precipitated by anger and disappointment, a struggle with "the mysterious incorporeal might of her anguish," she looks out of her window:

> Far off in the bending sky was the pearly light; and she felt the largeness of the world and the manifold wakings of men to labor and endurance. She was a part of that involuntary, palpitating life, and could neither look out on it from her luxurious shelter as a mere spectator, nor hide her eyes in selfish complaining.
> (Eliot, 1961, p. 750)

Eliot is clear that such an awakening promises "endurance". In Winnicott's terms, the move from object relating, with its hallucinatory promise, its mirages of the grand and the ideal, into object usage means coming to terms with being ordinary. This involves taking care and being cared for, as "labor and endurance" take their toll.

But there is also "the pearly light" to which Dorothea awakens. It is neither ethereal nor idealistic. She has been hurt, and this is the question she comes to: "What should I do – how should I act now, this very day if I could clutch my own pain, and compel it to silence, and think of those three!" (Eliot, 1961, p. 750). This is a form of surrender, unsheltered by the possibility of retreat, the glassy sheen of idealization or entitled demand and complaint. Just as the Skin Horse says, it hurts sometimes.

As therapists, we are given the unenviable task of persuading patients that their protected worlds of idealization and self-aggrandizement might be traded in for a life in which "most of your hair has been loved off, and your eyes drop out and you get loose in the joints and very shabby." What impels movement towards such a scuffed and scruffy modesty? Winnicott's answer is that the object-relating world without the brakes of negotiation and solid realness is terrifying in its intensity and muddle between inner and outer; that it creates insatiable gods and demons that need constant attention as early agonies beckon. Object usage brings perspective and obviates surprises.

There is something to be understood, however, about the potential of traumatic de-idealization to deaden the internal world. Access to fantasy is an essential part of potential space, and transitional objects are imbued with comforting qualities through being idealized. Without this imaginative, creative space, worlds of play and art, there is a danger that objects are reduced to things, material without life or depth. Winnicott insists on this paradox: the move from object relating to object usage, and its implied separation and engagement with concern and empathy, capacity to be alone (with someone), and the beginnings of the ability to conceive of multiple points of view, never implies that relationship is not always mingled with the affective rainbow and fantasies implicated in having an inner life. To stop at the outer door, without making up what lies behind it, is to be mind-blind (Allen and Fonagy, 2006). Further, it is projection, according to Winnicottian theory, that kindles a connection to an inner core, and, as importantly, convinces us that there is an inner core to be reached in another. Without this imagining, the outer walls are either just that, walls housing nothing, or worse, a crypt within which is entombed a dead connection. The trick is then managing projection as a source of creativity without it becoming densely distortive of the real world.

Notes

1 Issues with the use of the term "primitive" are taken up in Chapters 5 and 8.
2 For this insight and turn of phrase, I am indebted to Tony Frank, personal communication, May 2017.

References

Akhtar, S. (1996). "Someday . . . " and "if only . . . " fantasies: Pathological optimism and inordinate nostalgia as related forms of idealization. *Journal of the American Psychoanalytic Association*, *44*(3), 723–753.

Allen, J. G. and Fonagy, P. (Eds.) (2006). *The handbook of mentalization-based treatment*. John Wiley & Sons.

Bach, S. (1977). On the narcissistic state of consciousness. *The International Journal of Psycho-Analysis*, *58*, 209–233.

Bollas, C. (2013). *Being a character: Psychoanalysis and self experience*. Routledge.

Bromberg, P. M. (1983). The mirror and the mask: On narcissism and psychoanalytic growth. *Contemporary Psychoanalysis*, *19*(2), 359–387.

Eliot, G. (1961) *Middlemarch*. Zodiac Press.

Freud, S. (1914). On narcissism. *Standard Edition*, *14*, 67–102.

Gedo, J. E. (1975). Forms of idealization in the analytic transference. *Journal of the American Psychoanalytic Association*, *23*(3), 485–505.

Kernberg, O. F. (1974). Contrasting viewpoints regarding the nature and psychoanalytic treatment of narcissistic personalities: A preliminary communication. *Journal of the American Psychoanalytic Association*, *22*(2), 255–267.

Klein, M. (1940). Mourning and its relation to manic-depressive states. *The International Journal of Psycho-Analysis, 21*, 125–153.
Kohut, H. (1971). *The analysis of the self: A systematic approach to the psychoanalytic treatment of narcissistic personality disorders*. University of Chicago Press.
Mitchell, S. A. (1986). The wings of Icarus: Illusion and the problem of narcissism. *Contemporary Psychoanalysis, 22*(1), 107–132.
Slochower, J. (2011). Analytic idealizations and the disavowed: Winnicott, his patients, and us. *Psychoanalytic Dialogues, 21*(1), 3–21.
Slochower, J. (2013). *Holding and psychoanalysis: A relational perspective*. Routledge.
Spruiell, V. (1979). Freud's concepts of idealization. *Journal of the American Psychoanalytic Association, 27*(4), 777–791.
Stern, D. B. (2013). *Unformulated experience: From dissociation to imagination in psychoanalysis* (Vol. 8). Routledge.
Stern, S. (1994). Needed relationships and repeated relationships an integrated relational perspective. *Psychoanalytic Dialogues, 4*(3), 317–346.
Williams, M. (1922). *The velveteen rabbit*. Avon.
Winnicott, D. W. (1965). *The maturational processes and the facilitating environment: Studies in the theory of emotional development*. Karnac.
Winnicott, D. W. (1969). The use of an object. *The International Journal of Psycho-Analysis, 50*, 711–716.
Winnicott, D. W. (1989). *Psycho-analytic explorations*, ed. C. Winnicott, R. Shepherd and M. Davis. Karnac.
Winnicott, D. W. (2002). *Through paediatrics to psychoanalysis: Collected papers*. Karnac.
Woolf, V. (2017). *The essays of Virginia Woolf, Volume 5: 1929–1932*. Random House.

Chapter 3

Having a good peep

False selves and use of the therapeutic space

In Chapter 1, I described the ruthlessness of the fussy eater, the patient who quibbles over crumbs, turns down both delicate and hearty meals in the analytic space, and is then starved of nourishment. This chapter elaborates on this theme and complicates it in several ways. I will be suggesting that turning away from what the therapeutic space has to offer, while engaging the therapist in a ritual of offering and being spurned, week after week, is a ruthless defence that fully performs disengaged engagement in the way Guntrip (1992) has described. My particular interest in this defence relates to two other phenomena: Winnicott's description of the false self, and dissociative inability to connect in psychotherapy.

I have in mind a particular clinical presentation, in which the patient enjoys a full but secret relationship with the therapy. Everything said or done is stored and mulled over in a private space; the influence of the therapist on these private ruminations is hardly ever acknowledged, unless dismissively. As Khan suggested, there is also a pleasure taken by the patient in "having a good peep at himself" (Khan, 1960, p. 433).[1] In such a therapy, swathes of the patient's life might be unknown to the therapist, and sometimes changes for the better are only grudgingly admitted, in case they are consumed, attacked or spoiled in the sharing. There might be a continual private dialogue with the therapist, arguing points, elaborating or fantasizing a comforting exchange; these engagements, of course, are under the patient's control, and therefore protected from surprise or disappointment. But here is their danger too: in a system so closed to feedback, they fail to supply the kind of recognition that at some level is craved.

There are distinctions to be drawn between styles of self-presentation, all of which allow peeping without exposing a guarded and watchful interior. These include curated selves, which entail an artful and artefactual self-presentation, and bear a relationship to inner truths. There is also censorship, a presentation that leaves parts of the whole out of the picture, or play-acting or role-playing that may exaggerate or distort an inner truth. Then there is subterfuge, involving degrees of falsehood, and of course limited spontaneity, with glimpses of an inner way of being seen fleetingly like light seen through a thick panoply of leaves.

There are versions, seen from the outside, of self-presentation in peeping selves; so too is there variety in the mechanisms internally designing the peep itself. At the one end of the spectrum can be discerned a kind of hyper-mentalizing, a cautious pushing of the pause button before every answer, a quiet but determined accumulation of as full as possible a record of each interaction for later contemplation. In another version, there is room for some spontaneity in interaction, although the selves allowed into the public domain accommodate carefully to rules of engagement and setting. At the other end of the spectrum, an interacting self hides the fact of a relationship not only from interlocutors, but from full consciousness too. Here, there is no private dialogue or internal argument. Between sessions, the therapy is simply "known" but unthought about. In sessions, deadness might take over, an arid picking over of the events since the last meeting, with no projective enlivenment, no peep of curiosity, no galvanizing ripple of anxiety. Betty Joseph describes, for example, in her discussion of addiction to near-death, a patient who "seemed not to notice or be aware of almost anything about me as a human being" (Joseph, 1992, p. 452). Guntrip and Ogden suggest that such ruthless burying may extend to the patient's incapacity to dream, or even to surrender to sleep (Guntrip, 1992, p. 299; Ogden, 2003). Guntrip reports patients saying:

> "I fear I will never wake up again," or as one patient said: "I have to keep waking up at intervals to see how I'm getting on. It's so difficult going to sleep because it feels like going some place where there isn't anybody and you're really by yourself."
>
> (Guntrip, 1992, p. 300)

And yet the ritual of appearing for sessions is maintained, even as its futility seems to be underscored week after fruitless week. The patient has created a den, a retreat, beyond awareness, a bunker impenetrable to the nuclear explosions of connection (Bion, 1959).

The balance between what is secret and what is for public display will depend not only on setting, and a wide variety of factors unique to the individual, but also on social and political influences. The weight and potential threat of heightened affective involvement might make avoidance of shame, anxiety, envy or intimacy a priority, in ways that may have to do with historical or current trauma, early patterns of relationship, gender, class and culture, and personal idiom (Bollas, 2013).

That we all have access to different selves in interaction is a broadly accepted tenet of intersubjective and relational psychoanalysis, and indeed of postmodern thinking. Debates about what constitutes an interactive "core" and the relationship between multiple selves, dissociation and repression continue to be sources of contestation (Bromberg, 1995; Davies, 1998; Goldberg, 1987; Harris, 2011; Lachmann, 1996; Pizer, 1996). Exploration of the many meanings of dissociation has in the past two decades fundamentally reworked psychoanalytic ideas about the nature of the unconscious, and refocused analytic thinking on the place of trauma in structures of personality, after a long hiatus, during which the work of

Janet and Ferenczi were relegated to the back burner (Bornstein, 2013; Danielian and Gionotti, 2012). With the flowering of theoretical and clinical work on dissociation, its definition has sprawled (Bromberg 1996, 2013; Stern, 2010). For the purpose of this argument, I am making a distinction between multiplicity, with all its implications of potential for creative adaptation and spontaneous access to complex social and behavioural repertoires, and dissociation as a defence against, and sequestering of, painful affect and experience of trauma. While the former implies the capacity to lead a "full" life, the latter implies survival by dint of a psyche divided with no possibility of moving flexibly across compartments. Paradoxically, access to multiplicity of selves in health also implies an orchestrating and binding core, whereas a self divided into sequestered bits and pieces suggests the possibility of a weakened binding core, several seats of identity and potential conflict between them (Sinason, 2002).

Exploration of peeping selves suggests that there is merit in clarifying the distinction between multiplicity and dissociation both theoretically and clinically. Most broadly and simply, the term "dissociation" describes disconnected pieces. Again broadly, this disconnection might be between divergent selves, each with their own repertoire, a divide between unformulated experience and experience accessible to memory, the severing of affect from intellect, or very specifically, a walling out of trauma, frozen within moments in time and space. Disconnection suggests variable and patchy lines of communication between bits, and equally patchy access to conscious awareness of what is walled in and what is sequestered. The peeping self is different from dissociative phenomena in this respect: at its most developed, it admits a secret connection between bits and pieces. There is a layering of experience, a cautious harvesting to be collated in private, a bank of images and affects to be drawn on for rumination, art or donning of invisible hair shirts and whipping, instant replays of triumphs and blunders, and so on. Peeping selves might also have dissociative pockets of functioning.

It is a critical diagnostic concern to be able to map the extent to which dissociation in secret self-structures penetrates into and compromises accuracy of memory and access to a range of affect. If the trauma that led to the creation of a secret self in the first place is overlaid on object relating that relies heavily on psychic equivalence or pretend mode thinking, then what is culled from experience will be fragmented and infested with magic. I am positing, however, that a secret self might take root and flourish in a personality in other respects proficient as a mentalizer, and this offers psychoanalytic theory a unique opportunity to think through the relationships between dissociation, on the one hand, and secrecy, true and false selves, and their relationship to affect regulation and capacity to think, on the other.

It is worth contrasting the presentation of patients for whom a secret or private compartment, known or partly known to themselves, forms a substantial defence against psychic danger, with those for whom dissociation is a significant defence against affective storms. The latter are patients whose minds go blank in sessions, and who have patchy access to a continuity of being. The psychic splitting implicated in creating a secret self might be different in quality from dissociative splitting in the following ways. Dissociative patients "going blank" in sessions are struggling to articulate anxiety-laden material that becomes inaccessible in the moment: the wish to communicate it is not necessarily in doubt. Blankness involves the whole psyche-soma in a flood of disruption; there is no observing self "having a good peep" or squirrelling away material to contemplate at leisure. Moreover, there is no anaesthetized presentation of thoughts or events bereft of meaning. The dissociating patient is alive with meaning, and it is dread of its import that causes the emptying of the mind in the moment.

Secret selves spawned as a lifelong defence against relating are more likely to be connected to obsessional compartmentalization, creation of rigid in/out categories and watertight barricades than the fragmented and confused states of mind that overturn both memory and consciousness of dissociative patients. Dissociating patients seem to want to eat, but involuntarily deprive themselves of the means of doing so. Some patients with secret selves want to eat, but alone, and there they relish the food. Others wish to live on the thinnest gruel with which it is possible to sustain life. And some deny food by creating robots of themselves and the analytic process.

False/secret

Winnicott's descriptions of selfhood carry four centrally important notions for the purpose of this argument. First, the "true" self is the origin of the spontaneous gesture, creativity, a sense of being fully alive. From a self-psychological perspective, the self, when functioning cohesively, is flexibly independent, interdependent and a centre of initiative. In both Winnicott and Kohut, the true/virtual self is the space from which a developmental unfolding will proceed (Lichtenberg and Wolf, 1997). As Winnicott describes in "Metapsychological and Clinical Aspects of Regression," there are times when impingements require the nascent self to be "frozen in time"; the "unfreezing of the original failure situation" requires a regression so that development might begin again (Winnicott, 2002, p. 287; see also Kohut 1971; Newman, 2013). So both Winnicott and Kohut write of a core, authentic to itself, from which derives energy, zest for living and a will to create, rather than simply endure.

The second critical issue is that Winnicott's term "false" is misleading in one respect: he insists that a true self is "theoretical" in the sense that it can never be discovered, reflected on or lived into uncoloured by the many accommodations and ordinary injuries that being human entails. It is therefore possible to argue that the true self as a core of motivation and meaning, a source of desire and need, is folded into the unconscious. Critically, it needs *both* contact with *and* isolation from the potentially impinging spontaneous gestures of others. There needs also to be a growing capacity to tolerate multisidedness and ambiguity. Winnicott suggests in "Ego Distortion in Terms of True and False Self" that this is in the service of being able to "forgo omnipotence" (Winnicott, 1965, p. 143). If the true self must always be clothed to some degree in order to muddle through accommodation to living peacefully with others, the implication that this is not "true" needs complicating. It is perhaps useful to think of the adaptation of the true self to social living not as inauthenticity, but as flexibility. This includes a capacity to receive and generate new experience, but also to protect the self from difficulty, in ways that prevent fragmentation.

Third, to the extent that a false self comes into existence as a tactic to avoid the ambivalence, mourning and survival implicated in moving from object relating to object usage, it is always an amplification chamber for early anxieties, fuelled by fantasies of omnipotent control, on the one hand, and envious or greedy attacks on hoarded treasures, on the other.

Finally, it seems to me that Winnicott's classification of false self presentations brings into focus variations on the extent to which a true self may be accessible to the individual in question. At one extreme, Winnicott appears to posit conscious choice: "I will do this, in this social situation, as an acknowledgement of social rules, but my thoughts are my own"; at the other extreme, there are no "thoughts of my own." Here, a fully compliant, accommodating self-organization has been set up, and thoughts are those reflecting the unthinkable anxieties of others. The individual protecting a secret self is not necessarily protecting consciously a true self. There is a true self to be protected, as is generally true, but a vigorous defence is also mounted to protect parts of the self that lie between true and false, conscious and unconscious. Stubborn resistance to incorporation of secret compartments into communicative relationships prevents flexibility, but fends off colonization as well.

My exploration of secret selves needs to include some consideration of what "true" might be imagined to include. For Winnicott, this would certainly incorporate the capacity to be ruthless, in the struggle for survival, and this in turn involves zestful destruction of the object. From this, it is possible to postulate a true self that is both the originator of the spontaneous gesture but also of aggression and determination to triumph at any cost. The thread needs to be pursued a little further. Secret lives are led because for those harbouring them, there is fear of assaults of all kinds, from being colonized to being abandoned. Harsh criticism, humiliation and shame about vulnerability are all reasons to grow a carapace. The quest for the quality of the true self must then entail a question about the source of attacks on it. What is walled in and what is walled out?

According to Fairbairn, and Guntrip's humane and accessible amplification of Fairbairnian and Winnicottian object relations theory, sequestered parts of the self become echo chambers for apprehension of its capacity for destructiveness, either through love or hate (Fairbairn, 1994; Guntrip, 1992; Ogden, 2012). The extent to which attacks mounted within the self against the self can be considered projects driven by the true self is dependent on conceptions of basic human nature. For this argument, it is important to stress that a secret self is probably not complacent or lacking in conflict; on the contrary, and terrifyingly, it walls the enemy in, and builds a private amphitheatre for a ceaseless rehearsal of dreads (Akhtar, 2000).

Secrets, ruthlessness and ways beyond

In this chapter, I am arguing that the "engaged disengagement" of secret selves forms an effective (and ruthless) defence against a different kind of ruthlessness, one that allows for use of the therapeutic space to achieve nourishment. Provision in sessions might be drained of meaning, derided or unremarked upon, or may be squirrelled away for later contemplation. The idea of the peeping self also carries with it a promise of future availability, the deliciousness of hiding giving way to the delight and terror of at last being found (Winnicott, 1965, p. 186). At the same time, disguise in sessions is a dangerous business.

First of all, it misleads. The semiotics of the peep needs some further exploration here. Material brought as a decoy is always symbolically related to the concerns of the true self, however it disguises itself. For example, a patient might bring material that seems crisis-driven or richly elaborated in terms of links with past patterns, but these might not be central to the anxieties the private self is ruminating over. The danger here is threefold. First, for the therapist not to discern the difference between material offered as a subtle decoy and unspoken anxieties altogether unarticulated underscores the trauma of remaining hidden. Second, the material presented might be a decoy, and is narrated ruthlessly to lead the course of a session along one path rather than another, but nonetheless contains within it sufficient clues to prompt a search for an alternative route. Finally, peeping selves insert enough material into the flow of sessions to prompt enactments followed by ruptures that then serve as confirmation of the need for disguise of the most vulnerable parts of the self. In all cases, the peeping self is symbolized, and in a sense is fully present; it is this presence that allows the peeping. Being there in disguise, and not being seen, simply confirms the trauma that caused the splitting off into secrecy in the first place. Moreover, an attuned therapist will be aware, consciously or unconsciously, that clumsy attempts to link bits and pieces will cause painful vulnerability, criticism or withdrawal. The halt at the palisade therefore is by mutual agreement.

There is also danger in the ease with which attachment to the therapy might be overlooked. As Betty Joseph points out, "The analyst seems to be the only person in the room who is actively concerned about change, about progress, about development, as if all the active parts of the patient have been projected into the analyst" (Joseph, 1992, p. 454). If the therapist acts to end the therapy, believing it to have run its time, this may cause a devastating injury to the hidden parts of the patient who never declared his or her affiliation openly.

In these ways, failure to recognize the secret self, however fleetingly it appears, is a profound repetition of the calamity that caused the original secrecy to become a way of life. To the extent that disguises carry vulnerable parts of a hidden self, they carry filaments of self-display, and to brush them aside is a dismaying and shaming injury. In the act of peeping, the patient's self is under scrutiny behind a veil, and unthinkable anxieties are stirred, with no possibility that they might be properly received and understood. This reinforces the individual's conviction that self-soothing and holding things together is doomed to be utterly solitary; it increases a sense of futility in trying to communicate; and it makes putting the brakes on anxiety very difficult. Here, the fact that object relating rather than object usage is in play is critical.

At the same time, seeing what has not been freely offered for sighting places the therapist in the role of predator or voyeur, in itself an impingement.

Finally, some consideration needs to be given to the other secret self in the room. It is part of the psychoanalytic contract that therapists have private selves, and depending on the branch of theory that they practice, this extends to all details of their personal lives, and at least partly to what they think as therapeutic sessions are under way. Some of these thoughts are shared, with both tact and compassion being valued as essential to successful communication. There is general agreement that "sharing" of class, culture, personal taste (clothing, choice of furniture) and even political beliefs is inevitable, as markers of all these are clearly imprinted on body and setting. There is also a demand that therapists, within the bounds of tact and compassion, are truth-tellers, and in line with this, that they bring at least a version of a true self – a self in which authenticity is felt and to be trusted – to all treatments. The extent to which these factors are in play has occasioned lively debate (Corpt, 2013; Mitchell, 2014; Orange, 2002), and will continue to do so while major differences with respect to transference interpretation remain.

For the purpose of this argument, the private self of the therapist remains foundational to the provision of a setting in which the patient takes centre stage as subject. Further, the therapist's capacity to use reverie depends on periods of interactional disengagement. Part of the patient's unfolding as subject results from establishment of potential space, in which the capacity to be alone when needed and without fear of impingement is critical. If the therapist is able to maintain authenticity while preserving safe space for reverie, this will be both guide and bulwark for the patient, a place of tethering and mutually protected engaged disengagement.

There is one respect in which the automatically assumed secret self of the therapist may become a complicating factor in a therapy with a peeping self. There are two parts to this. It is not always the case that secretive patients are adept at spotting the therapist's self-displays consciously, but they are often unusually sensitive to inauthenticity (McWilliams, 2006). So, the therapist's juggling of multiplicity with a patient who juggles with disguise is a recipe for muddle, misrecognition and rupture. In addition to this, there will always be an extent to which the therapist's secret or sequestered selves are kept within strict limits while a session is taking place, but are available for hijack by material half-hidden or disguised in the peeping patient's dense elusiveness.

This all suggests that therapies with patients who are secretive will require the therapist to be unusually deft in a number of ways. There must be capacity – or an act of faith – to imagine a growing bond with the therapeutic project, despite tenuous evidence of connection. This needs to be married to listening laterally, in order to make links that the patient has made every possible conscious effort to disguise. The self allowed fleetingly into the therapeutic space must be seen and recognized just enough not to be alarming. Playful engagement with disguise, subterfuge, irony and paradox might well be important in creating the therapy as potential space for trying on the experience of show-and-tell, without the stakes being too high (Coen, 2005). Finally, McWilliams suggests that "the willingness of the analyst to be 'real' – to be flawed, wrong, mad, insecure, struggling, alive, excited, authentic – may be the most believable route to fostering the schizoid person's self-acceptance" (McWilliams, 2006, p. 20).

Tickets to the peep show: the curator

She had a glossy head of hair, carefully and yet casually arranged. Had I known to look, there was the whole thing: immaculate disarray, the paradox with which we would wrestle for years. Her clothes elaborated on the theme: they were carefully selected, outfit by outfit, to be at once cohesive and suggestive of nonchalance. Paradoxically, she presented spontaneity, with the hours of craft behind each presentation carefully erased. I mistook the performance for a bold assertion of individuality, a comfort with self-expression, and this took the therapy down an alluring, but blind, alley.

She was senior in her profession and worked with severely traumatized people. She had a reputation for both reliability and warmth. Her ability to cleave through to the core of a problem, and to saturate murky corners with light, led to a series of professional successes. She worked for long hours and took on more and more responsibility. The burden of expectation that she continue to create miracles led to increasing anxiety, a pattern of being susceptible to migraine, and a growing sense that unless she agreed to every demand, she would find herself jobless. She felt in some respects like a fraud. Again, in retrospect, her initial presentation of her difficulties paradoxically told everything: she was right that her performance of total, warm presence in the service of others was always a partial truth, and promised a whole self, when only a small part was visible.

I was told of all these anxieties as if she was living through them with me in the sessions, but the cohesiveness of her narrative, absence of strong affect as she recounted particular situations, cheerful accommodation to my interpretations, and an eerie sense that we were both being spectators to a play hinted at the untold and unshared.

There were ebbs and flows to her social life. For many months, she would see few people socially, apart from frail parents who lived near to her, and with whom she had a pleasant but enmeshed relationship, and siblings with whom she had occasional contact. When she was in a romantic relationship, she would be embraced by the partner's friendship circle and would have times of being socially very active. Her tendency to hide her opinions and needs, both with partners and their friends, often left her feeling unseen and unattended to.

Sessions were filled with enlivening commentary about her work. This was linked sometimes with her sense of anxiety that she would over time fail to meet people's expectations. She would describe an interaction with a colleague; it would be coherent and deliciously full of irony, but also coloured with resentment about the burden she carried, and attacks on herself about her inability to provide everyone with perfect advice. Unprompted, she would consider many points of view, and would also take care to reassure me that our work together was helpful to her.

The familiar shape of sessions changed during the times of having a romantic partner. She would then spend time thinking about her experience of ambivalence. She would want to fold herself into the life of the partner, to share living space and to do everything together, but she also felt anxious about giving up her solitude and being engulfed by someone else's needs. Caught between fear of being abandoned to a life alone and fear of being consumed and erased by a relationship, she frequently chose connection, at least for a time. She would also find herself participating superficially in all aspects of the relationship, but keeping her thoughts and needs strictly to herself.

That there was a secret self having a peep became apparent very slowly. For example, I would sometimes be told about the impact of a comment I had made months before. She would sometimes report in a session on progress made on a problem shared many sessions before, and in rich detail would inform me of the ways in which she had used our work together to think it through and find a way forward. Over time, it became clear that she curated the material brought to sessions, containing the problem before sharing it with me, and then using our interaction privately. In this way, she and I were able to put our heads together over a self never entirely in the room.

Despite peeps, despite enjoyment of this woman's seductively self-deprecating and witty stories, sessions became more and more difficult to see through to the end of the hour. I found myself wondering why the curator kept coming. At the same time, she carelessly announced her times of travel for business and her vacations. I could see ways in which she had used the therapy effectively, but continued to worry about her levels of stress, long hours at work, and the effects on her health of the levels of trauma she encountered daily. My sense of estrangement from her, and the apparent desiccation of the exchanges between us, needed to be discussed.

What followed surprised me, and was further evidence of the extent to which she had sequestered her feelings about the therapy to an internal world that she could visit at will, and alone. She became tearful as soon as I enquired about her sense of the therapy and its usefulness to her. She apologized for uneven attendance and assured me that her time with me was essential to her ability to manage her life. She became anxious when I tried to deepen this exploration, and quickly moved the session on to curated ground.

Shortly after this unfolded, a crisis broke open the rhythm of the sessions, and for a time I felt I had access to her lived experience, as it was being lived. Romantically involved with a colleague whom she discovered was using drugs, she was for a time unable to make a clear boundary between work and home. The colleague-turned-partner became enraged as she withdrew, and was convinced that she was pursuing relationships with other men. There were many arguments, and on two occasions these had ended sharply as a result of threats of physical violence and rape.

For the duration of this crisis, the curator was able to access material not only about the current situation, but also about its links to a childhood in which she was subjected to ruthlessly demanding treatment by her parents. It felt as though an entirely new phase of the therapy had begun, and that we would now be able to immerse ourselves not only in memory, but in reverie steeped in affect. It seemed that this might begin to coax a secret self into a trustful relationship, and the possibility of using the therapeutic space ruthlessly, to meet her needs rather than to keep me at bay. As the crisis receded, however, she also slipped back into her seclusion, and the etiolated connection began again.

For many months after the crisis had passed, and the curator was settled again into a solitary life, I was told about ways in which she thought about what had happened, and conclusions she had come to as a result of these private ruminations. I was witness to a process that seemed productive and satisfying to her. Her reports to me seemed to be about assuring me that there was lively and independent internal life that I was trusted to see from a distance. It was also an act of compliance. That she reported on her thoughts as belonging to the past was the act of curation; the spontaneous spilling out of thoughts as they occurred to her in the present was not yet a possibility. In this sense, the therapy was not a transitional space, a place of play, and she was unable to use it ruthlessly, to receive the affective acknowledgement, collision in meeting and the survival she needed to explore its full possibilities. It was nonetheless ruthless in defending the part of herself that needed to be sequestered. The time lag became more striking as the therapy progressed: she could discuss almost any topic with me so long as she had turned it into a spectacle, an exhibition we could both view from a distance. In this way, we came to understand that the self kept secret from me was the one experiencing in the moment, having thoughts, and holding those for later contemplation.

The pattern of contemplation, then curation, then presentation to me changed in small incremental steps over many sessions, during which the curator worried that she was simply repeating herself (Bloch, 2009). The sense of the present being held hostage by curation, and of both past and present looping in a way that drained each of meaning, was interrupted gradually in two ways. First, a second relationship crisis, accompanied by fierce waves of anxiety, allowed her to bring a distressed and spontaneous self into the space. The links of this crisis with her family history became a foundation for occasional access to affective pockets during periods in which her life was relatively routine. Second, she became involved with outdoor adventures such as hang-gliding and white-water rafting that filled her in the moment with adrenalin and enabled her to come to sessions full of excitement. My obvious pleasure in hearing about her exploits brought a spontaneity to our interchanges, and this began to build a bridge between inner and outer worlds, the secret and the displayed.

The accountant

He had organized his life so that very little feedback trickled in. He did his work in a methodical way, and although it often felt routine there was some satisfaction in its tidiness. The hours were long, and he maintained an amiable persona with colleagues, who regularly asked him to take the lead with complicated accounts. At home, he lived a busy life in parallel to his wife. At times, he would resent the ways in which he was made to feel responsible for keeping the home in a functional routine. Mostly, he retreated into a world of books and music, cut off from intimacy, and alarmed at interruption. He consulted me during a time when he was wrestling with futility, his work increasingly drained of purpose, and with a struggle to calm himself at night.

He was unable to use the therapy space to dream with me, to enter reverie, to bring a self in need of being seen. He did react powerfully, however, to being welcomed in. In his alarm at the spotlight, and the implicit request to talk freely, he found a way of tying us both into a version of intimacy: he drew me into abstract statements about art, life and meaningless – these hinted at a depth of suffering that made me deeply concerned. As I tried to explore his place in the abstractions, there would be more abstract statements, until I felt I was no longer following the conversation at all. I was left with a single link between us: my own growing wish to reach the part of his self that had been sequestered, and was showing itself in this disguise, and the appeal that he transmitted when he glanced my way.

He told me that he often thought about the sessions when on his own. He had fantasies in which he and I had the conversations hinted at but never embarked on in the sessions. He made it clear that these conversations accompanied every part of his day, but he gave me no hint as to their substance. The apparent intensity of his focus on me, and his vigorous private use of me, seemed to provide rich material for analysis, but when I tried to follow associations I met more abstraction. I came to understand this intense and paradoxically unshared intimacy as a kind of addiction, enlivening for him, but also anaesthetizing him against the pain of bringing his affective needs into interaction with me. Moreover, in elaborating the conversation between us in fantasy, he was able to feel that he was taking a good peep at me. This perverse use of ruthlessness to avoid ruthless use of the therapy time had us locked into a disconcerting performance of intimacy that hinted at its presence while simultaneously keeping it in the wings.

The accountant was punishing himself for his lack of joy, his dying ambitions, his loneliness. He felt resentful of the ways in which his own sense of order and financial acumen seemed to give his family permission to be disruptive and careless with resources. He sometimes mentioned feeling guilty about his internal dialogues with me. Despite this guilt, his readiness to report on them suggested some energy invested in putting me on the spot. I was presented therefore with a coyness in his account of the many conversations he imagined us into. We both became spectators to the conversation that had happened offstage.

Over time, I was offered occasional opportunities beyond the mists of abstraction to "play" with what I might have said or thought. Initial explorations, including his associations to various ways in which he placed us as interlocutors, and his fantasies about what I might say and why. This allowed me gradually greater access to "flawed, wrong, mad, insecure, struggling, alive, excited, authentic" realness. On one occasion, we improvised an imagined conversation he had with me about solitude in the time between sessions, and this absurd and ironic riff set in motion new playfulness and levels of attunement between our embodied selves (Knoblauch, 2013). My interjections made him laugh and put him at ease; they also reassured him about the extent to which I was entering his world, and playing alongside, if not with, him.

Voyeurism and food

A senior colleague once suggested to me that a self having a good peep hauls the carcass of the session off to a cave to devour it in private (Stephen Bloch, personal communication, 2017). In our discussion, we amplified on this metaphor to include the idea of tokens kept after crimes of violence. There are overtones, of course, of sacrificial meals. He reminded me that in writing about psychotherapy, we too are feeding on the nutrients gifted to us by our patients, and often after they are "dead to us," either because they have terminated therapy or been so disguised that they are wraiths of their former selves. It is completely true that as therapists, we are always witnessing our patients' lives, with permission, and they are peeping into ours: just as they glean information from our taste in cushions and pot plants, so we pick up information about when to plant out seedlings and where to buy excellent used cars.

When Winnicott suggested that we want to be eaten, however, he had in mind something very far from secret eating, and from a cannibalistic ritual too. What is being attacked and destroyed are the anxieties that lead to secrecy in the first place. Psychoanalytic theorists writing on patients with schizoid defences agree that these patients often have a tormenting or tormented inner world, in which a choir of critical or persecutory voices constantly inhibits spontaneity. Amplifying those voices in the therapy involves torment at first, but as they are heard and spoken back to the table can be laid for a shared and truly nourishing meal.

Note

1 Masud Khan's reputation has been tarnished by his ethical infractions both as an analyst and as a writer; nonetheless, his writing on private selves retains pockets of deeply resonant phrases.

References

Akhtar, S. (2000). *Broken structures: Severe personality disorders and their treatment.* Jason Aronson.

Bion, W. (1959). Attacks on linking. *The International Journal of Psycho-Analysis, 40,* 308–315.

Bloch, S. (2009). Music and the dreaming of absence. In *Cape Town 2007-Journeys, Encounters: Clinical, Communal, Cultural: Proceedings of the 17th Congress of the International Association for Analytical Psychology*. Daimon, 251–259.

Bollas, C. (2013). *Being a character: Psychoanalysis and self experience*. Routledge.

Bornstein, M. (2013). Dissociation and repression: A clinical study. *Psychoanalytic Inquiry*, *33*(5), 439–448.

Bromberg, P. M. (1995). Psychoanalysis, dissociation, and personality organization: Reflections on Peter Goldberg's essay. *Psychoanalytic Dialogues*, *5*(3), 511–528.

Bromberg, P. M. (1996). Standing in the spaces: The multiplicity of self and the psychoanalytic relationship. *Contemporary Psychoanalysis*, *32*(4), 509–535.

Bromberg, P. M. (2013). *Awakening the dreamer: Clinical journeys*. Routledge.

Coen, S. J. (2005). How to play with patients who would rather remain remote. *Journal of the American Psychoanalytic Association*, *53*(3), 811–834.

Corpt, E. A. (2013). Peasant in the analyst's chair: Reflections, personal and otherwise, on class and the forming of an analytic identity. *International Journal of Psychoanalytic Self Psychology*, *8*(1), 52–69.

Danielian, J. and Gionotti, P. (2012). *Listening with purpose: Entry points into shame and vulnerability*. Jason Aronson.

Davies, J. M. (1998). Multiple perspectives on multiplicity. *Psychoanalytic Dialogues*, *8*(2), 195–206.

Fairbairn, W. R. D. (1994). *Psychoanalytic studies of the personality*. Psychology Press.

Goldberg, P. (1987). The role of distractions in the maintenance of dissociative mental states. *The International Journal of Psychoanalysis*, *68*, 511–524.

Guntrip, H. (1992). *Schizoid phenomena, object relations and the self*. Karnac.

Harris, A. E. (2011). The relational tradition: Landscape and canon. *Journal of the American Psychoanalytic Association*, *59*(4), 701–736.

Joseph, B. (1992). Psychic change: Some perspectives. *International Journal of Psycho-Analysis*, *73*, 237–243.

Khan, M. (1960). Clinical aspects of the schizoid personality: Affects and technique. *International Journal of Psycho-Analysis*, *41*, 430–436.

Knoblauch, S. H. (2013). *The musical edge of therapeutic dialogue*. Routledge.

Kohut, H. (1971). *The analysis of the self: A systematic approach to the psychoanalytic treatment of narcissistic personality disorders*. University of Chicago Press.

Lachmann, F. M. (1996). How many selves make a person? *Contemporary Psychoanalysis*, *32*(4), 595–614.

Lichtenberg, J. D. and Wolf, E. (1997). General principles of self psychology: A position statement. *Journal of the American Psychoanalytic Association*, *45*(2), 531–543.

McWilliams, N. (2006). Some thoughts about schizoid dynamics. *Psychoanalytic Review*, *93*(1), 1–24

Mitchell, S. A. (2014). *Influence and autonomy in psychoanalysis*. Routledge.

Newman, K. M. (2013). A more usable Winnicott. *Psychoanalytic Inquiry*, *33*(1), 59–68.

Ogden, T. H. (2003). On not being able to dream. *The International Journal of Psychoanalysis*, *84*(1), 17–30.

Ogden, T. H. (2012). *Creative readings: Essays on seminal analytic works*. Routledge.

Orange, D. M. (2002). There is no outside: Empathy and authenticity in psychoanalytic process. *Psychoanalytic Psychology*, *19*(4), 686–700.

Pizer, S. A. (1996). The distributed self: Introduction to symposium on "The Multiplicity of Self and Analytic Technique." Contemporary Psychoanalysis, *32*(4), 499–507.

Sinason, V. (Ed.) (2002). *Attachment, trauma and multiplicity: Working with dissociative identity disorder*. Psychology Press.

Stern, D. B. (2010). *Partners in thought: Working with unformulated experience, dissociation, and enactment*. Routledge.

Winnicott, D. W. (1965). *The maturational processes and the facilitating environment: Studies in the theory of emotional development*. Karnac.

Winnicott, D. W. (2002). *Through paediatrics to psychoanalysis: Collected Papers*. Karnac.

Chapter 4

The weeping couch

Universities in South Africa are in trouble. In this, they are not dissimilar to universities worldwide. There are major questions of financial viability, with rising staff costs, the need to keep afloat through student fees and research grants, the substantial burden of keeping campuses serviced and maintained, the demand to protect researchers' time from the demands of large undergraduate classes, and a desire to creep up the world rankings in order to attract both international students and research projects. On top of these global pressures, there are local difficulties, complex mixes of economic, political and social forces to which universities must respond, to avoid stagnation, irrelevance, and moral and financial bankruptcy (Jansen, 2017).

Responses to the demand that universities reinvent themselves as flexible, solvent, and responsive to local and global, economic and political realities are very varied. In some scenarios, specialization is the route taken, with institutions choosing to concentrate their resources in science, the arts, medicine or engineering. Some focus on postgraduates, others on providing basic tertiary education at relatively modest cost to students. Some keep staff salaries low in order to preserve a degree of open access for students who would otherwise not be able to afford university education; some depend heavily on a long history of wealth, accruing through bequests, property and donations from alumni. Industry plays a role in feeding money into professional training programmes and research projects from which they might benefit. However they manage to balance the books, universities are seldom profit-making institutions, even during an era in which having tertiary education is a key factor in ensuring stable employment and upward mobility.

Pressures on universities are changing their character fundamentally. They cannot remain spaces of privilege for the wealthy and connected; nor can they maintain a lofty ideal of being a playground for thought, creativity, experiment and invention. The "absent-minded professor," lost in thought, buried in an office littered with papers covered with arcane scribbles, will only be tolerated if the output, measured in papers published, grants earned, Nobel Prizes won, warrants it. Armies of relatively poorly paid contract lecturers and tutors, micromanaged through systems of surveillance and feedback, come and go, with little prospect of finding a permanent berth in academic employment. Diversity in the student intake in terms of class, race, culture, gender and preparedness for university provokes the need for new teaching technologies. Exponential change in knowledge boundaries and its web-based dissemination demands that curricula reshape themselves year by year.

The mix is volatile and undoubtedly creative. One function of the university as a social institution has not changed at all: it is the space in which generations of young people become excited about ideas, take risks, and plunge into the task of reading, writing and making knowledge their own, shouldering aside their scholarly elders and daring to dream of originality. No wonder, then, that universities are often the spaces within which social and political upheaval ferments and amplifies, where manifestos are written, and protests foreshadow broad social demands for change. As Maldonado-Torres points out, it is the gathering together of youth, in whom hope for the future is invested, and who feel fundamentally opposed to being positioned as "sanctioning the present order and continuing its existence in the future," that makes centres of learning "important zones of struggle"(Maldonado-Torres, 2016, p. 2).

The university from which this case study is drawn, the University of Cape Town, is a hybrid institution, combining large undergraduate numbers and a strategic plan that emphasizes its "research-led" status. It has a creditable world ranking in terms of the QS World University Rankings, respectable research output, and many postgraduate and professional training programmes with excellent international reputations. It has property in prime positions and an impressive plant. Despite all this, the balance between staff salaries and fee income has required management to institute austerity measures, such as leaving empty posts unfilled and trimming back on course offerings. Of course, ways of implementing austerity measures, and even the degree to which management is being transparent about the need for austerity, are constantly contested by both staff and student bodies. Long perceived, with some justification, despite a modest history of anti-apartheid struggle, as a bastion of white privilege, UCT, along with other South African universities, has faced several years of student protests, the effect of which has been fundamentally transformative. Change has been demanded ruthlessly, and it has come.

The protests constellate around three major issues: the need to decolonize structures, space, knowledges, social engagement and institutional culture; the need for free education, or at least a lowering of student fees; and the need to reverse a past decision to outsource service workers such as cleaners, kitchen staff and maintenance crew. These three pillars of struggle are central to the decolonial struggle in the following ways: they question international criteria for measuring scholarly excellence through mechanisms such as rankings; they insist on access to free education as fundamental to societal transformation; and they foreground workers' rights as implicated in overturning habitual forms of privilege (Maldonado-Torres, 2016). The term "decolonial" in this context signals striving for change more far-reaching than the material, governmental and power hierarchies implied by decolonization: critical is its reach into structures of both knowledge and subjectivity.

The background to the student protests in South Africa has been a sluggish economy, rising levels of unemployment, growing poverty, increasing evidence of corruption in government, gender-based violence on a massive scale, and a significant burden of illness with thin provision of healthcare infrastructure for those without means to access private resources. In the course of the protests, there has been disruption to the academic programme with times of total shutdown, precipitating unprecedented attention to matters of student fees, student accommodation, artworks displayed across campus, committee membership and lines of institutional accountability to stakeholders, curricula, and workers' contracts.

My experience of different aspects of this transformation is described in this chapter, and also in Chapters 5, 6 and 7 (see also Bosch, 2017; Nyamnjoh, 2016). The focus of this chapter is on the arrival of institutional turbulence as a result of student and worker protest. It describes turbulence arising from ruthless demand on the institution as object, and the destruction/survival cycle that it sets in motion. The period described is located in the eye of the storm, during the collision with the object, in the hallucinatory world of object relating, before object usage is achieved (Winnicott, 1969). It will explore local effects on ordinary going-on-being within individuals, each negotiating their own relationship to the ruthless demand. It also broadens this frame of reference to consider ruthlessness, destruction and survival in the working of standing committees attending to routine academic, student and staffing business, such as registration for courses, uploading of marks, payments to departments, release of funding for research, and examinations. It tries to make sense of how organizational turbulence spreads outwards, through institutional structures, as well as inwards, into the emotional lives of the individuals who animate those structures. It looks at the ways in which a demand that an institution reexamine its habits, taken-for-granted membranes of object relating that have held a particular fantasy of itself together, disrupts work, causing deferrals and interruptions, and creates the need for emergency decision-making and new regulations.

The intersection between a protest movement, the executive response to it and the working of local committees is complex, and turbulence in one arena cannot simply be mapped on to the bumpy trajectory of another: each has its own dynamic, set of defensive manoeuvres, strategic goals, deadlines and urgencies to attend to. Psychoanalytic thinking has a contribution to make in understanding this interface, both in terms of understanding its overt systems of operation and its underlying largely unconscious anxieties, where more perverse forms of ruthlessness are frequently deployed. These student protests I describe serve as an example of decolonial struggle. More broadly, my analysis in this chapter is focused on ruptured interfaces that protest movements create between the ordinary and the ongoing, and necessary shifts in the management of time, space and subjectivities no longer contained by routine. Further, organizational rupture has a relationship to individual trauma, and each amplifies the other.

I am interested in the difference between "turbulence" and "trouble" in this context (Fischer, 2012). Fischer makes the helpful distinction between turbulence as an organizational characteristic and trouble as having its roots within the dynamics of particular individuals. This chapter will trace the trajectories back and forth between turbulence and trouble. In doing so, it will raise issues about how psychoanalysis might approach distinctions between individual and group processes. The role played by ruthlessness in search of recognition in both turbulence and trouble will be a critical focus. The chapter will begin with common assumptions both in the psychoanalytic literature and in lay knowledges about the unconscious life of a group in volatile conditions. It will offer a case study of a committee affected by organizational turbulence, and will illustrate an instance in which individual trouble, intersecting with constant impingement from unprecedented institutional change, changed the form and direction of critical decisions. Perverse ruthlessness and the dangers of local corruption during situations of turbulence will be explored. The chapter will end with some thoughts about the meaning of organizational survival during ruthless attack, and possibilities of collective mourning in its aftermath.

Turbulence and trouble

Fischer (2012) makes a distinction between "trouble" in a system constellated around the relational difficulties of an individual, and "turbulence," which disturbs the routine functioning of a whole system. Turbulence might originate in the relational trouble of an individual and those immediately in the path of its stirring, but the local contaminates and reverberates, taking advantage of the system's connectedness, one part with another. Fischer describes the way in which "what begins as localized trouble tends to create emotional contagion, stimulating further trouble elsewhere in the community" (Fischer, 2012, p. 1161).

Trouble is ubiquitous in all organizations, and in fact has the important function of underscoring the need for rule-governed behavior. Trouble easily becomes narrativized as a moral tale, demonstrating to the collective what happens when rules are broken. The literature suggests that organizations might deal with trouble as private or even confidential; however, leakiness in relational boundaries ensures that transgressions become "known," sometimes in distorted and forbidding forms, totems against further mad or bad behavior (Fischer, 2012). As one past deputy vice chancellor at the University of Cape Town acerbically announced, the only way to keep anything confidential was to pin it on a noticeboard. Paradoxically, it is the injunction of maintaining confidentially in isolating "trouble" that ensures its currency as "news." It seems that dealing with trouble "behind closed doors" is functional as a form of boundary policing with multiple tasks. It establishes hierarchies of police, judges and juries in a "privy council." It closes the door on those without standing in the matter, communicating that there is something of grave concern afoot. Trouble also creates an occasion for rehearsing the rules (if not the particular infraction) in public gatherings. In short, it serves the system as a highly efficient way of foregrounding general rule-boundedness and apparent transparency.

Drawing on Winnicott's idea of potential space, Fischer suggests that trouble might create a liminal space within which a system finds creative ways to transform. By definition, trouble throws the rules up into the air, and the "play" of setting everything to rights offers the opportunity for relational spaces to be restructured. Most particularly, the phantom monsters hidden behind rules are briefly toyed with, and then packed away, and the anxiety accompanying their appearance is for a while a little less compelling.

Fischer also suggests that turbulence reverberating within a system independent of localized trouble might be creative in affirming its larger purpose, offering opportunities for clarifying and polishing boundaries and ways of communicating. Shaking loose expectations of how things are "always done" and experimenting with the unfamiliar, the apparently risky or transgressive renews roles within systems and provides opportunities for networks of relationships to cohere, using local attachments as cement while scaffolding new structures. He also points to the possibility that both trouble and turbulence might take a perverse course, driven, for example, by resistance to change, refusal to participate in opening potential space, or using uncontained destructiveness to repeat the system's current and past traumatic patterns.

Relational connectedness in systems suggests that trouble, unless quickly contained, will reverberate beyond the troubled individual; similarly, turbulence will trigger trouble through stirring up local relational difficulties. Words such as "contamination," "infection" or "taint" are frequently used to describe the reverberation, suggesting the invisible passage of a disease through the corporate body (Wallace, 2007). The analogy works well: communication of trouble and turbulence implies an exchange, person to person, of a common disorder, resulting in feverishness. This must not be confused, however, with superstitious or magical accounts of transmission, as each microbial event is traceable relationally between people, and historically through the durability of DNA in the form of role expectations over time (Chapman and Long, 2009).

The interlocking roles of trouble and turbulence can be illustrated with the following brief example. Imagine trouble accumulates around the person of a single lecturer running one compulsory undergraduate course on a difficult topic that challenges the boundaries of students' willingness to read complex material. The students ask for a slower pace and easier assignments. He digs in his heels and refuses to adapt any part of his course, claiming the students are lazy and reluctant to put in sufficient groundwork to comprehend the material. He becomes irritable in and out of lectures, and loses his temper with both administrators and tutors working with him. Two of them are seen, at different times, crying in the corridor. A sympathetic young lecturer gives comfort, and in her office there is a cushioned "crying chair" in frequent use. The lecturer withdraws from social engagement with colleagues, and there is staff tearoom talk as his students complain in various other courses and among each other about their grievances. Before long, trouble that was confined in one week to the boundaries of a single course is extended through another trouble generator, a student who feels the department as a whole is unresponsive to student feedback. Although apparently this view is not widely held, it is nonetheless taken up and broadcast by students from various courses, all of whom have struggled, or anticipate with dread the upcoming struggle, with the problematic compulsory course. Soon, the structure and sequencing of the department's courses, including that some are compulsory and others not, become the eye of the storm. Trouble has now tipped over into turbulence, petitions are circulated, lectures boycotted and the department's levees are breached as news reaches the dean that an intervention will be required.

A creative solution to the turbulence would probably involve a series of meetings, an acknowledgement of the students' real anxieties about difficult compulsory courses, a reflection among staff on the department's course structures and content, and a "behind closed doors" discussion with the original source of the trouble, leading perhaps to some modification of his expectation and methods of teaching and examining. One can also imagine a perverse route: the staff meet and declare the students "illiterate," "underprepared" and "lazy"; *they* had to read at this level when they were undergraduates, so why should this generation not have to do so? The original trouble source was "right to take a stand." In this, the staff is bolstered by the attitude of a distracted but narcissistic head, stung by criticism, but too busy with research projects to invest time in knot-unravelling. The opportunity to be creative is gone, and in defending itself against perceived attack the department ensures that it will garner a reputation for being unsympathetic to students' needs. This rumbles through every new intake, friends passing on to friends the reputation of "killer courses" and arrogant lecturers. The cycle repeats.

Mapping the complex connections between trouble and turbulence allows analysis to take account of individual histories of success and failure, trauma and habit; it also obviates the need to imagine systems as having minds of their own. Groups are potentially sites of emotional contagion, especially in affectively charged situations. To the extent that individuals within them subsume their personal identities to the imperatives of the group's goals and needs, there might be pressure to sacrifice multiple points of view in order to see contradiction or ambiguity. In this way, turbulence affects deeply all individuals within a system, foreclosing on some paths of thinking, and rolling out others as "obvious" or "unavoidable." When turbulence involves threat to the system itself – to habitual ways of doing things, for example, or to its assumptions about the environment within which it operates – then anxiety is heightened. Importantly, it is not the system that is anxious, but individuals within the system, and for some this brings to the surface individual vulnerabilities. As individuals resonate, this in turn reverberates through the system, a vicious circle that binds individuals and groups into turbulent cycles.

The view of group dynamics as ruthlessly compelling compliance in ways that operate outside of individual conscious awareness was the basis of Le Bon's influential work on groups, and was elaborated in Freud's "Group Psychology and the Analysis of the Ego" (Freud, 1921; Le Bon, 1897). As Freud pointed out, there is a great deal of evidence that individuals will sometimes behave in groups in ways that would be completely foreign to them in other contexts. At the same time, the trouble and turbulence argument suggests that individual dynamics might coerce groups into similarly foreign ways of behaving. Inspiring leaders have just such an effect. In some systems, a perverse dynamic, set up by an individual enlivened by chaos, for example, or recreating an environment of disorganized attachment, might trigger turbulence in a vulnerable system. It is to examples of this that the argument now turns.

Turbulence at the University of Cape Town

The kinds of trouble and turbulence on campuses in South Africa are linked to a demand for fundamental change to both the systems in place and the subjectivities of those working within them. They have this in common with the goals of protest movements everywhere. It is with the experience of alienation of black students, staff and workers, and the rupture that brought with it the frightening, luminous possibilities of new ways of being, that this account is primarily concerned.

As Winnicott suggested in his work on transition from object relating to object usage, ruthlessness serves as a statement, a challenge to the object, an assertion of difference and differentiation, a demand to be taken seriously as an actor with agency. In the course of the collision, a dependent, undifferentiated self is lost. In its place, there is a new way of being. The complexity of the moment of rupture separating two modes of being is that it is both ordained – in the sense of being inevitable – and yet faces everyone with a future that cannot be predicted and may involve a slide back into repetition of a past that refuses to be destroyed.

In the first instance, need for systemic change constellated around the Rhodes Must Fall movement, described in more detail in Chapter 6. The foregrounding of black students' experience of alienation on campuses has shaped the students' protests as fundamentally a demand for recognition in the terms Fanon (1986) describes. The protests were highly effective in creating turbulence. The rupture was decisive. Students' occupation of the university's administrative building inserted the protest into the university's engine room, and as ordinary routines sputtered and then fell silent, the stage was set for a new beginning. The halters of old were thrown aside. Over the next 18 months, the university hobbled through closures, revised timetables, new scrutiny of rules, fees, hiring practices and provision of services. There were times when a mirage of the old appeared – for some a welcome familiarity, for others a spur to further action. There were long meetings, negotiations and sometimes violence. Students' demands began to be addressed with variable success. For this accounting, it is the dramatic shift in subjectivity that the turbulence produced that I will now describe.

The flowering of a new awareness was not subtle and is traceable to the ordinary arteries through which the blood of an institution flows. For example, roles on critical committees changed, along with their membership. The status of old guardians of time immemorial slipped into verdigris. Familiar items on agendas were replaced with new ones speaking of emergencies and risks and transformation; student leadership in meetings was approached with anxious solemnity. New rules quickly found their way into the books, bypassing laborious debate and delay. Rules of debate also changed. In the face of visceral challenge, affectively heightened by angry accusations and expression of trauma, well-rehearsed master narratives crumbled. Some previously authoritative speakers fell silent, resonant new voices filled the halls. "Privilege" had none of its old currency; in short, we had a new economy. What some had thought of as gold turned out to be of dubious worth.

My description suggests a kind of cohesion that misrepresents the messy reality. Individuals came and went in their habitation of new roles. Groups that were ranged against each other in the conflict dug themselves in from time to time, each accusing the other of betrayal and lying. For some, the conflict seemed to become a way of life, not a means to an end. The silence of some sectors hid resentment rather than sober reflection. There were times when there was deep confusion about the kind of recognition the protest movement required. None of these contradictions negate the sea change in atmosphere, the newness of the landscape through which we moved.

The rapidity of the change also brought anxiety and exposure of trauma with histories linked back into childhood. Dismantling privilege as it nestled in universities' long histories of "tradition," in the case of UCT squarely linked to colonial ties still evident in buildings, values, degree structures, and curricula, with those of Britain, the "mother country," brought both irritability and dissociation. A radiating web of defences tied all irrevocably to old fault lines. Recognition of the new and survival of the collisions it inevitably brought about with what was "traditional" was always going to be accompanied by rehearsals of old forms of being and blindnesses, the pain caused by old institutional routines. Some of these took the form of individual troubles, which I describe in the following section. At UCT, there was a collective series of enactments, a parade of defences, many not subtle. In the midst of turbulence, "business-as-usual" meetings were sometimes held, as if nothing had happened, as if protesters were not shouting outside the door. Slips of the tongue infested public statements, resulting in retractions and clarifications. Hope and dread washed back and forth like waves and backwash, making it hard to see the movements of tides, and they brought every defence one can imagine: wild optimism and grandiosity, denial, dissociation and narcissistic rage. All of us were vulnerable to trouble.

Trouble

During the 2015–2016 period, I attended hundreds of hours of meetings, some of them standing committees, some emergency gatherings to deal specifically with the protests. The "trouble" I describe here flowed out of the organizational turbulence in which we were embedded. I have disguised detail to protect the confidentiality of both the committee and the individuals between whom the interaction took place.

The interaction did not stand out as unique in any way, and I use it to illustrate the ways in which subjectivities access both broader intersubjective fields and the cobbles and coils of individual dilemmas to produce moments of heat and repetition of trauma, as well as opportunities for hope. The example I use here concerns a committee and academic staff, and the dynamic it illustrates is relevant to the complex ways in which turbulence and trouble interact. Although it played out in response to protest action, it is intended to illustrate a general dynamic. Later chapters will address the decolonial dynamic specifically in greater detail.

As so often in moments of crisis, the knot presented itself as a funding issue. A group of students with a high profile in the protests needed both free accommodation for several weeks and extra tuition for classes missed. This required permissions up the hierarchy to move money from one fund to another. In this particular committee, some members guarding the budget and trying to balance the books in extraordinary times insisted that the funds were simply not available. The decision to fund or not to fund is never simple, but at this stage in the conversation no one seemed to have a personal stake in it. All acknowledged, on the one hand, scarce resources and, on the other, the political imperative to meet the students' need. The conversation began its first circle of the table.

One man, Professor X, previously an outspoken supporter of the students' demands, voiced his dismay at the way in which the cost of hiring extra accommodation had escalated over the period of a month. He also expressed his irritation at the "recalcitrance" of some staff, not on the committee, refusing to be flexible about offering students in need both accommodation and the extra classes and opportunity to submit assignments during the university long vacation. At the same time, he made it clear that the threat of chaos if the students' demands were not met made him feel cornered. He became animated as he spoke, insisting that the committee chair find a way to broach the urgency of the students' needs with those in the university hierarchy. He held contradictory views, common in informal talk, but for the purposes of this case study it was a significant signal of a subjectivity undergoing a sea change. On the one hand, he was expressing irritation with a university hierarchy he found unsympathetic to the students' plight. On the other, his experience of the students' ruthlessness as threatening a structure, routines and his own survival as a mediator made him turn to the university's parental authorities with a ruthless demand of his own. He wanted "the committee" to cut through impediments, make provision exactly as the students demanded, and for the crisis to be averted.

Then another committee member, Professor Y, began to go over the history of the request for funding. She claimed to have a memory of the original, more modest request, detailing the numbers of students to be accommodated, a much smaller number than the current one. While she was elaborating, a little pedantically, on her understanding of a deal brokered some weeks before with representatives of the student movement, Professor X became heated, repeatedly interrupting her account with mounting impatience. An awkward silence gave way to a hiccup of surprise and hurt from the interrupted Professor Y. After a little time, and with tears in her eyes, she gathered her papers and left the room. For a few moments, the committee was silent. Then it was suggested that the decision about the students' request be deferred until more information had been collected.

The radiating coils of this interaction mirror both the broader turbulence and the ways in which it might trigger individual trouble, which then feeds back into turbulence. I turn now to what happened with the passing of time.

Professor Y did not, in the short term, survive this cycle of conflict, this destruction without repair. She had been a supporter of the student movement, and felt misrecognized by Professor X's implicit accusation that she was insisting on a strategy that would be harmful to individual student leaders. However, it actualized a visceral fear of feeling, in her words, as she recalled the incident later, "unwanted," a sense of her position in family and school hierarchies with which she had lived since childhood. Neglect had made her both an ambassador for the neglected and sensitive when feeling her thoughts were being unattended to. Unable to brush off the interaction and move on, she resigned from the committee, saying she no longer felt able to contribute meaningfully to its work. In this way, she created a painful re-enactment of the sense she carried with her of being always in the process of being cast aside. Her breakdown had already happened, but her choice of institutional setting made its rehearsal inevitable (Winnicott, 1989). Professor Y collapsed into what appeared to be a kind of falling forever, a going to bits and pieces in that space, which was then cemented by her bodily and mental withdrawal. Seeking affirmation, especially diffidently, from committees in bureaucracies is a risky strategy.

There is another part to this story of the intersection between trauma and a wider context of organizational turbulence. Professor Y might have been susceptible to being wounded in any committee, in any year, but I would argue that the layers of conflict in the university context imported amplified stress and irritability into many meetings. A sense of urgency infected decision-making processes and truncated leisurely discussion. That there was urgency was indisputable, but in the case of Professor Y, already reverberating with anxiety resulting from her wish to represent that which was being put aside, being spoken over, somewhat roughly, confirmed the trauma residual to parental failure to affirm her.

Professor X seemed outwardly to survive, but not to thrive. It emerged that he had made promises to students and to persistent staff fighting the students' cause in informal meetings with respect to availability of funding, assurances he desperately wished to honour. These promises were not his to give, and he feared that his credibility on the committee and with the students would be undermined. After his rageful intervention, he retreated into a glowering silence in meetings, interjecting only when rising anxiety led him to fend off imaginary accusations against him. For example, when criticisms of the committee's decisions surfaced, he would say, "So I suppose Person A or Group B thinks *I* did that." It was precisely this sense of persecution, and attempts to appease attacking forces, that had caused the trouble in the first place. He remained an unhelpfully hyper-vigilant committee member, fending off enemies from all sides, and the scratchiness of this ensured that he would be vulnerable to exactly the distrustful scrutiny he feared others were turning on him. For him, too, there was a complex intersection with the turbulent context. Torn as he was by persecutory anxiety, going to war with an enemy clearly defined and in his sights gave him a temporary sense of safety, but this was always undone by the fantasies of revenge being taken against him. The way in which Professor X invested the student protesters with the power to retaliate, and make an assault on his reputation, if promises he made were not upheld also speaks to this.

The splitting of good from bad, and here the projection into "management" and "protesters" of destructive impulses, was heightened by the rhetoric of the protests, which was explicitly threatening from time to time. Inevitably, the ways in which Professor X waged war made such vengefulness in those cast into the enemy camp more likely. The way in which this pattern of behavior was repeated through various committees and several months of meetings suggested it was not a temporary state of mind, but one exacerbated by tumult, and leading to serial enactments, all traumatizing in their effect.

The relational matrix of the committee, too, seemed not to survive, in two senses. First, members were unable to hold and reflect on the conflict that had erupted in a way that considered the welfare of all, choosing a dissociative defense to avoid conflict and to defuse heightened affect. Second, members also deferred the committee's work, leaving the dilemma that had caused the conflict unresolved. An appearance was maintained of moving through the agenda, of a gathering into a mask of professional exchange, but this was to be one of many instances of deferral. In spite of a wish to meet students' demands, members of the committee ended up not doing so, which then fed into a broader perception of the institution's sluggishness and resistance to change.

The committee's failure to survive represented a hollowing out of itself, the basis for which speaks also to splitting and projection. While Professor X's attack on Professor Y was regarded with distaste by members of the committee, many of whom communicated this in sidebars to meetings, he nonetheless gave voice to a common set of fears: of being identified as "management," and therefore as "against" the student demands, and beneath that of playing into the kind of organizational resistance that would result in victimizing particular groups of students, and further disruption to the university's programme. This was a committee generally known to be strongly supportive of the university's need to change, and yet the disarray caused by one set of sentences uttered in anger points to a layer of fear, not unlike Professor Y's: of being found to be "unwanted" and dispatched to a space of irrelevance, an organizational death. Winnicott would perhaps describe this as a reaction to impingement that results in introversion, a protection of an inner world safe from an environment that has in fantasy become entirely persecutory (Winnicott, 2002, p. 208).

It is in this way that enactment shadows a broader dynamic and folds itself into anxieties that rippled through the institution as a whole. It is not incidental that the event was gendered, and embodied one aspect of the students' explicit agenda, the need to address aggressions and microaggressions against women, nor that the dispute was triggered by funding and accommodation, both of which were protest pillars. So, every layer was folded into every other, receding hallucinatory mirrors, leading not through, but round. At every point, there was ruthless defence, not a breaking through, but a breaking down and a breaking in, enabling early anxieties to take hold.

Ruthlessness and rupture

This local failure to thrive raises its intersection with the broader dynamic in which it was encapsulated. In what ways might local failure echo through the whirlwind spirals of institutional life in turmoil? There can be no definitive answer to this, and much will depend on the complex ways in which individuals and groups, protected by defences and bolstered by a collective will to recognize multiplicity, weather each tornado. That being said, I want to follow this case study through to its next iteration, and to use both Winnicott and Fanon to suggest that to see this example of collapse into repetition as an ending does less than justice to an outcome that carries strands of hope for a new pattern.

In "Aggression in Relation to Emotional Development," Winnicott argues that "aggressive impulses do not give any satisfactory experience unless there is opposition" (Winnicott, 2002, p. 215). The opposition comes from the environment, and sets up the possibility of collision, which in turn establishes a not-me reality. In this context, opposition is an affirmation of impact, and is essential to being recognized as a separate centre of initiative. He suggests – and this is the bedrock of Jessica Benjamin's position too – that perfect adaptation to angry demand must include both recognition and opposition: to cave in does not allow full expression of aggression, while total opposition leads to either withdrawal or cycles of violence (Benjamin, 2017). Just as Fanon suggests, too, freedom cannot be conferred, as conferring simply perpetuates a relationship of unequal power.

It is against this backdrop that the workings of the committee might be read. On the level of the two individuals involved, there was a collision, a collapse and a withdrawal. The immediate effect on the committee was dissociation. It would, however, be short-sighted to end the interpretation there.

It was of paramount importance that the students' needs momentarily brought the committee's deliberations to a halt. At every level of the university, such moments took place, and each one marked rupture with the past. It was in each of these bruising encounters that individuals became other than themselves. Second, even though the committee deferred making a decision on the occasion of that meeting, like the environment-mother, it held a space in time, and set in motion the possibility of a future response. By default, it also avoided collapsing into a demand, by holding a position that spoke, however faintly, of the possibility of compromise and a range of provisions. Finally, I believe that the expression of aggression in a committee whose membership excluded students brought outside turbulence inside, and unpleasant though the moment was, it bridged a divide between two worlds of affect, an impossible opposition between calm business and fiery cataclysm. The penetration of the one world into the other established change as both me and not-me, as real, with neither side "mere things" (Fanon, 1986).

Conclusion: the weeping couch

In Winnicott's view, it is survival of ruthless attack that opens the way for an experience of concern, the capacity to see through the eyes of the other, to acknowledge difference. For Melanie Klein (1940), it is reaching the depressive position, embracing the ambiguity of living in relationship, and the good and bad that tempers the impact of each unmutated. In Russell's (2006) terms, it is the delivery of grief. For an institution in crisis, moving beyond a collectively held sense of persecution, with armies ranged against each other, towards ease with juggling complexity, will signal survival.

The movement from ruthless challenge to mourning, and in the case of this protest movement to finding security in having finally broken through the dehumanization of a colonial situation, raises a specific set of issues in universities. For example, for a university to mourn for a past steeped in colonial privilege is both impossible and inappropriate. Moreover, there is a sense of sure-footedness needed by a transformed institution, and while universities globally face such uncertainty, we shape-shift in ways that make grief rites difficult, particularly as they require being able to imagine a future space in time. However, using the example of my committee once again, in my experience there is a patchy, piece-by-piece way forward that holds individuals' grief as the institution lumbers its way beneath them. It gets encapsulated in gestures of care and in angry clashes that end in a murmured "Oh, I can see that." New people in old roles and old people in new roles stumble and reach out for help, across ideological divides. Most importantly, change itself becomes ordinary, familiar, a way of living that incorporates the routine and the banal.

The web of connections between individual trouble and institutional turbulence becomes critical to understand in this context. The constant thread of trauma repeated, from which recovery will be slow, provides impetus for change; it also carries a threat of dissolution, of everything falling to pieces. My argument in this chapter has been that trauma will always be registered singly and specifically in the bodies of individuals, as it was with the professors in the case study described above. The burden of the repetition is theirs to bear. However, trauma is not isolated within the body of an individual: it communicates beyond itself. There, it generates resonance, and becomes constellated as a signifier for a class of traumatic experiences, and will be carried through turbulence into a tipping point of change. In a decolonial struggle, it is this that needs some further thought.

My focus in this chapter has been on the broad strokes of a dynamic that links individual trouble with institutional turbulence. I have not therefore been specific about the ways in which individuals involved in decolonial protest action carry a burden of trauma that constantly threatens survival and must claim the fight for survival not as an individual right, need or desire, but as a claim to be humanized. It is not simply a struggle to surf the trouble-trauma waves that might throw some individuals back into their earliest encounters with misrecognition. It is a struggle for breath in the "metaphysical catastrophe" of being regarded as subhuman (Maldonado-Torres, 2016, p. 13). In the colonial situation, and a decolonial struggle, there is "endless war on specific bodies, cultures, knowledges, nature and peoples," and, as Maldonado-Torres succinctly puts it, "bodies bleed" (Maldonado-Torres, 2016, p. 4). The metaphysical catastrophe is deepened suddenly, and in ways that threaten continuity, by exposure to the possibility of (in Winnicott's terms) having a true self, and simultaneously having this true self threatened with attack. In "Ego Distortion in Terms of True and False Self,"

Winnicott suggests that it is precisely these moments that heighten the risk of suicide as an avoidance of further unbearable exploitation (Winnicott, 1965). It is for this reason that survival of turbulence in a decolonial struggle will founder without generous resourcing of services to provide for specific bodies, bleeding with specific incursions on the ability to draw breath.

Maldonado-Torres maps ways in which coloniality "perpetuates itself through multiple forms of deception and confusion" (Maldonado-Torres, 2016, p. 2). For example, there might be institutional responses to the demand for "urgent" change that reconfigure space, change rule books and adjust the composition of committees, but that nonetheless continue to underwrite the privilege of northern hemisphere knowledges through scholarly partnerships, use of technologies that exclude some student sectors, or more simply and fundamentally allow attributes of "graduateness" to remain unchallenged. It is certainly true that institutions change slowly, with frustrating ebbs and flows. It is also true that coloniality, with its embedded master/slave dynamic, reinvents itself with disheartening obduracy, not only in societies scarred by colonialism, but all situations of institutionalized inequality. However, this makes the endeavour to measure real gains, and to chart the progress of change, where it has happened, all the more urgent. Gains are sometimes undramatic, consisting of no more than quiet moments of reflection, acknowledgement of both change and shame, mapping of complexity, guilt, small triumphs, complicity.

There is one other fundamental issue to be raised in relation to the case study I have offered in this chapter. It concerns the anthropomorphism of attributing affect to organizational structures.

For Winnicott, holding a space in time is a quality of survival. It is not solid, and is only holding because it is not imbued with "thingness." Holding a space in time is distinct from the timelessness of fantasy. It allows memory, experience of change and future possibility. It is impersonal, in that it is a space into which actors must move. In that it allows time, it is infused with idiosyncratic meaning. Most importantly, it constitutes the dimension within which differing points of view collide and reach for recognition. It contains the endless acts internally produced.

Committees at every level of my institution, and in my experience of many other institutions, have formal or informal terms of reference, designated meeting rooms and rules governing ways of speaking. They hold a space in time partly through the idea of rule-boundedness, however much particular rules change in response to challenge. They are also holding spaces through forms Winnicott, in "Metapsychological and Clinical Aspects of Regression," would attribute to "setting" in psychoanalysis: routines established over time of method, a tempo, attention to bodily comfort, adequate lighting, injunctions against interruption, and so on (Winnicott, 2002). It is in this sense that a committee holds a space in time – in Winnicottian terms, a potential space.

Committees are sometimes experienced as ruthless in the ways that they trundle on as membership changes and context transforms, with the weeping outside the door seemingly unattended to or not heard. But committees are rooms with rules. Just as the couch does not weep, committees as structures do not grieve. Nonetheless, they contain an atmosphere, they transmit affect around the table, and in the ruthlessness of their being "just" a space in time they carry the capacity to hold a regression and to entertain hate. They are therefore essential to the delivery of grief.

References

Benjamin, J. (2017). *Beyond doer and done to: Recognition theory, intersubjectivity and the third.* Routledge.

Bosch, T. (2017). Twitter activism and youth in South Africa: The case of #RhodesMustFall. *Information, Communication & Society, 20*, 221–232.

Chapman, J. and Long, S. (2009). Role contamination: Is the poison in the person or the bottle? *Socio-Analysis, 11*, 53–66.

Fanon, F. (1986). *Black skin, white masks*. Pluto Press.

Fischer, M. D. (2012). Organizational turbulence, trouble and trauma: Theorizing the collapse of a mental health setting. *Organization Studies, 33*, 1153–1173.

Freud, S. (1921). Group psychology and the analysis of the ego. *The standard edition of the complete psychological works of Sigmund Freud, Volume XVIII (1920–1922): Beyond the pleasure principle, group psychology and other works*. Hogarth Press.

Jansen, J. (2017). *As by fire: The end of the South African university*. Tafelberg.

Klein, M. (1940). Mourning and its relation to manic-depressive states. *The International Journal of Psycho-Analysis, 21*, 125–153.

Le Bon, G. (1897). *The crowd: A study of the popular mind.* Fischer.

Maldonado-Torres, N. (2016). *Outline of ten theses on coloniality and decoloniality*. Fondation Frantz Fanon.

Nyamnjoh, F. (2016). *#RhodesMustFall: Nibbling at resilient colonialism in South Africa*. Langaa.

Russell, P. L. (2006). The negotiation of affect. *Contemporary Psychoanalysis, 42*, 621–636.

Wallace, E. M. (2007). Losing a training analyst for ethical violations: A candidate's perspective. *The International Journal of Psycho-Analysis, 88*, 1275–1288.

Winnicott, D. W. (1965). *The maturational processes and the facilitating environment: Studies in the theory of emotional development*. Karnac.

Winnicott, D. W. (1969). The use of an object. *The International Journal of Psycho-Analysis, 50*, 711–716.

Winnicott, D. W. (1989). *Psycho-analytic explorations*, ed. C. Winnicott, R. Shepherd and M. Davis. Karnac.

Winnicott, D. W. (2002). *Through paediatrics to psychoanalysis: Collected papers*. Karnac.

Chapter 5

Masks, slipping

What characterizes the link between protest movements and potential emergence of lasting intersubjective change? In particular, are there connections between ruthlessness, rupture and the decolonization of consciousness? These are the questions with which this chapter is concerned.

The question of fees affordable for students whose parents are not in the middle class is at issue immediately when questions are raised about the ways in which institutions reproduce the lines of privilege associated with the colonial past. The struggle for decolonization is a struggle for material change, through redistribution of wealth and institutional power. There can be no doubt that such material changes, in conjunction with investment in public health systems, housing and education, would effect transformation and enable a move away from a visible and traumatizing cushion of privilege, colonial in origin (Long, 2018). The decolonial project incorporates decolonization, but goes further. In Mignolo's words:

> The decolonial turn is the opening and the freedom from the thinking and the forms of living (economies-other, political theories-other), the cleansing of the coloniality of being and of knowledge; the de-linking from the spell of the rhetoric of modernity, from its imperial imaginary articulated in the rhetoric of democracy.
>
> (Mignolo, 2011, p. 48)

Its "epistemic disobedience" reaches into basic assumptions privileged under conditions of coloniality (such as definitions of what constitutes knowledge or the technologies that contribute to constructions of "fact"). Decoloniality requires a rupture with an assumed natural order, and with it new forms of subjectivity. It seeks to rehumanize a world divided through hierarchies of difference by "the production of counter-discourses, counter-knowledges, counter-creative acts, and counter-practices that seek to dismantle coloniality" (Maldonado-Torres, 2016, p. 10).

In the argument that follows in this chapter, I will assume, as Long (2018) and Hartman (2005) suggest, that material change in social environments is deeply implicated in psychological change; this is a substantive part of decolonization. Decolonizing consciousness might be scaffolded in some ways by changing material conditions, but requires more than this to unseat prejudice long in the making: it is a project of decoloniality. My focus will be on the forms this demand for a change in consciousness might take. In particular, the chapter will describe the internal disjunctions and the ruptures in consciousness that interrupt familiar ways of being and ready the ground for new awareness. I will argue that protest movements offer a way of penetrating into dissociated and alienated states that form an initial bulwark against change. They create a kind of doubleness, identifications across boundaries, fissures in familiar roles and rules. Disruption of this, always accompanied by pain, lends itself to waking, and psychoanalytic theory has a contribution to make in understanding the process.

Protest movements, wherever they occur, are blunt, sloganizing and othering of the opposition. They tend not to deal in nuance or contradiction; negotiation and the tolerance of multiple perspectives may come only after gains have been made, and after the conditions for a shared reality have been negotiated and tested (Winnicott, 1969). Public protests at their most strident by necessity signal their presence loudly. They are embodied energetically and sometimes become wild. Their rhetoric splits good from bad, undoing reason in making sometimes impossible demands, and being therefore "irrational." They dream a new landscape, hold something or someone to ransom. Occasionally, in their ruthlessness, they become violent, tearing apart structures that represent their foe. In defying habitual routines, assaulting received wisdoms and ignoring decrees from authorities, protests reveal social contracts for what they are: a shared illusion, which is replaceable by another illusion.

Protests in South African universities will be used here as a case study to illustrate ways in which transformations of consciousness might be traced. Through social media, staff and students in conversation, and shared academic programmes and publications, the South African decolonial movement has had ties to global movements, with allies including Black Lives Matter in the United States and the worldwide #MeToo revelations.

Protests in South African universities have the prohibitive cost of tertiary education for the country's majority as a central focus. Along with the demand that fees must fall, protesters have insisted on a national conversation about the need to decolonize South African universities by freeing them from what is seen as enslavement to northern hemisphere knowledges. These are embedded in curricula often very similar to those taught in the United Kingdom or the United States, with too little acknowledgement of local context (Mamdani, 2018). To decolonize the curriculum might involve, for example, illustrating mechanical engineering theory with application to local challenges, weighing African and European literatures equally without treating some as part of a classical canon and some as exotic and other, and immersing health science students in the kinds of social, linguistic and medical skills that will enable them to apprehend the complicated intersections between class, culture, gender and the burden of disease. There are also rituals and rigmaroles – paraphernalia caught in bits and pieces of rule, art and habit – that continue to mark an allegiance to a colonial history seemingly remembered fondly by those with wealth and privilege (Bosch, 2017; Jansen, 2017; Nyamnjoh, 2016). Some examples of the rigmaroles are easily jettisoned: the singing of *Gaudeamus Igatur* before the slow capping of graduands at graduation ceremonies is an example. It is more difficult to think through the ways in which degree structures, rules articulating links between committees, and the balance between academic and management skill might be implicated in the decolonial project.

The decolonial movement is complex and affects every layer of an organization, from its ways of presenting itself to the public through to its innermost and hidden machinery. It is about dismantling the material and subjective markers of an oppressive past, embedded in a society scarred by race, class and gender division. As Wahbie Long puts it, we are being asked to look squarely at the "lived realities of ordinary South Africans, realities that are embedded in a landscape soaked in ableism, classism, gender-based violence, and racial humiliation" (Long, 2017a, p. 307). It is a landscape, a still-colonized world, in which "*everyone* is alienated, *all* are implicated – including us as psychotherapists who attempt to disalienate ourselves through our work" (Long, 2017b, p. 84, emphasis in original).

Alienation brings otherness as a long and inescapable shadow. Those with privilege – mobility, ownership of property, the luxury of access to voice – are living in a world in which dissociation from always-present deprivation and suffering is a way of life, an unthinking habit that fractures consciousness. For those struggling with material and emotional survival, there is the double consciousness of wretchedness and being seen through the eyes of the other as wretched (DuBois, 1989; Fanon, 1986). Both ways of splitting consciousness – being half-sentient or being made to be double – shatters cohesion. Fanon suggests that "being-for-itself" without doubleness, the seeing self as other, being beside oneself, "can be achieved only through conflict and through the risk that conflict implies" (Fanon, 1986, p. 218). This chapter explores conflict and its effect on consciousness as one part of the decolonial project. It draws its material from South Africa, but speaks to struggles against oppression and alienation wherever they are found.[1]

Being blown to smithereens

The trajectory through beginning to wake up from a consciousness that has sequestered its own privilege, or walled off awareness of alienation, shut down its own capacity to abrade and make raw, or determinedly sealed sources of self-esteem off from the appraising eyes of the privileged few is cumulative and necessarily painful. It requires a shift in an identity, often alongside a set of values and moral beliefs holding the meaning of who may pass judgement on whom, and the weight and place of ubiquitous concepts such as "being helpful" or "paying attention." I describe here moments of being jolted into a beginning of wakefulness, a state constantly in the making. In *The Wretched of the Earth*, Fanon talks of a "clear image . . . within the grasp and imagination of every colonized subject . . . to blow the colonial world to smithereens" (Fanon, 2004, p. 37). I describe here examples of the process of subjectivities being blown up internally, moments in which those inhabiting privilege are forced to change, but also those resisting continuing oppression bear the force internally of an explosion both sought and dreaded. With these examples as background, I will then look to theory to make some sense of the explosion.

The examples that follow describe the contours of encounters I witnessed in the course of one period during the height of the 2015 university closure. In each one, the shattering of an old order became embodied through micro-moments of testimony, accusation and counter-accusation. That the individuals speaking were deeply affected was plainly visible, and the sombre mood of the watching groups signalled the impact of what was being seen. There are two points to be made about this: that confrontation with urgent need to inhabit new forms of consciousness for those positioned as privileged and gatekeepers was accompanied by both fear and fragmentation, and that those speaking up against their colonization were being asked to revisit and perform the trauma of which they spoke. The terrible cost of putting aside a mask, of refusing double consciousness, was clear, as was the shaming display of privilege dismantled.

In this narrative of subjectivities both fluid and fixed, I begin with a set of enactments that embodied themselves in ownership of space as an emblem both of colonial occupation and of its reappropriation in the course of the protests. Its effects provided a perspective on the subjectivities of those involved, and the ways in which the identities of each side hardened the height of one wave of protest.

At the time that students were attempting to enforce the campus closure by disrupting lectures and urging staff to close their offices and go home, it became a practice in some buildings for staff to work behind locked office doors. This led to a cat-and-mouse game, with students listening for the tap of keyboards, and then banging fiercely on the door of the working staff member until he or she emerged and left for home. The confrontations played out in these circumstances were often experienced as frightening for those behind the locked door. The fantasy that had brought them to position the protesters as physically dangerous was fed by the shouting, banging and apparent threat of a break-in. For their part, students, being positioned as dangerous, but also having their call for a shutdown defied, were encouraged to redouble their efforts to empty buildings through implied threat and noise.

The behaviour of staff varied strikingly from building to building. In some, working behind locked doors seemed to become expected behavior, and information quickly passed between staff members about when the protesters were going to do their rounds. As the noise approached, staff would turn off lights, close blinds and sit in silence for the moment to pass. In other buildings, staff would readily move out of their offices and talk to each other or to protesters on the avenues, some signalling solidarity with the cause, some seeking information and some thoughtfully witnessing the ongoing events.

During this period, it was suggested that staff avoid hiding behind locked doors, as this seemed likely to increase the trauma of those hiding, and to provoke protesters into physically insisting on doors being opened. This message was received in a variety of ways. There were men expressing rage at their rights being infringed, and the university failing to protect their health and safety, their academic freedom. They insisted that as custodians of the academic project, contained in their research and teaching, they would not be bullied into submission. This expression of resistance to the demands of protesters was coming quite literally from behind a barricade. Women staff seemed more in touch with fear of physical assault, but also with the needs of their departments and students to do urgent planning, paperwork and administration despite their sense of the risk to themselves. In this way, there was a gender differentiation in subjectivity, even in the group behind the barricades. On the other side, there was a sorrowing in some protesters at those staff insisting on working in their offices. Shaking his head, one said that the constant battle across the barricades was simply wasting time that should be spent on negotiating beyond the shutdown. In one angry foyer encounter, a protester and an angry student objecting to being told to leave the building resulted in a brief physical struggle. It was a woman in the band of protesters who pulled the pair apart and took her furious comrade aside to try to prevent a widening fracas.

That ownership of the building space became an eye of the storm in a decolonial struggle is not incidental; neither were the hardening of attitudes on both sides. The fight was literally over a place to call home, and the right to do what one wanted in that space, challenged by those who claimed that ownership of space was a means to refuse the kinds of change they hoped for. I turn next to a situation in which subjective change, rather than crystallization into complementarity, is a focus.

With a small team of staff trusted by protesting students keeping watch and mediating from time to time, one department held a meeting at which they attempted to come to grips with practices that students characterized as traumatizing and saturated in white privilege. These included approaches to teaching, curricula, hiring policies, comments made on assignments, and availability of staff for supervisory consultations. On the face of this, every issue raised was easily remedied. It was, however, the flow of acknowledgement back and forth, the embodiment of a history of traumatic exclusions for black students, and a witnessing of shame-saturated realization of damage done that was primary. The adjustment to everyday practices would need to follow. The meeting began slowly, and anxiety mounted in the room. One lecturer, who had been singled out as being problematic for black students because of the ways that she offered them guidance in a form they experienced as patronizing, began to address the meeting. She started with an apology for causing pain, and she labelled this as inadvertent. She then went on to describe how she saw the protests, and how much she was in support of the need for change. In doing this, she assumed both that the protesters would welcome her support and that her summary of the state of play would chime with theirs. Even if it had, in the moment, this would have been an appropriation, a colonization of a struggle that could only be explicated from within, by those who owned it. Her apology then enacted the privilege against which the students railed.

It triggered a dramatic reaction in several of the student activists, one of whom began to cry loudly. She left the room, and for a time the group broke into discomforted clumps, some wondering whether it was worth trying to continue the meeting. It was a moment of being blown up.

The lecturer at the centre of this dramatic unravelling was at first angry, and then seemed bewildered by the effect her words had on the student. Soon after, she retreated tearfully to a chair in the corner of the room. The crying student was comforted by friends, given a cup of tea and eventually rejoined the circle.

This interchange was powerful in its effects. It enacted precisely the kind of blind patronage and lack of conscious awareness of casual othering of which the students complained. It triggered an outburst that revealed the depths of trauma experienced silently by black students who felt they could not be part of the university community as themselves, but only as visitors being prompted by staff to become something else, to disavow their identity, to consolidate their disappearance behind an acceptable mask. Finally, it seemed to have the effect of marking a way forward for everyone in the room, sending each one into an internal adjudication, identifying with one or other of the interacting pair, and considering the volcanic implications of speaking. For some, coming to understand what had happened in those few minutes would begin a process of change in consciousness. For others, there was comfort in the ruthless destruction of the group's habitual way of moulding events to old narrative paths.

Survival and repair was, however, still in question. In the aftermath of this meeting, some were concerned that though it had been intended to air grievances and heal wounds, it seemed only to have inflamed them. For a time, there was a retreat. Then there was a smaller gathering, attended by some student representatives and selected staff, to talk about practical details of trying to bring the academic year to a close. There was stout bargaining on both sides, and it seems in retrospect that this was one moment in which object relating, with all its clouds of projection, its fuel of fantasy and terror of murdering and being murdered, segued into object usage, adorned with lists and timelines for both sides.

That a shift had taken place was captured in an exchange that was both prosaic and exquisitely representative of the shifting subjectivities with which all were wrestling. The staff had arrived with tea, milk and biscuits. Both students and staff offered to make the tea and serve it. The students made clear that this was their domain, and staff were to have tea conferred upon them. This was not an act of servitude, but of hosting, the difference being made clear by orders issued. And with this simple ritual, a new going-on-being was instated.

The grappling with subjective change encapsulated in confrontations directly between protesters and staff or management also unfolded in interactions less directly about the protests themselves. They did, however, have an impact on decolonizing consciousness and the acknowledgement of black pain. The following is a narrative that illustrates ways in which managing moments of crisis is amplified by the waves of protest. In the course of a night of protest meetings, one student was reported to have followed another into a storeroom, apparently with the aim of touching her against her wishes. Neither student was centrally involved in the movement, but both had attended the meeting. The woman involved reported the incident to staff and protocol had been followed, but the traumatic event quickly became emblematic of allegations that the university was careless around procedures in cases of reported sexual harassment, unresponsive to black pain, and invested in protecting patriarchal interests. The alleged perpetrator added to the conflagration by making public accusations against the student he was supposed to have pursued. There was disagreement among staff about ways of dealing with the situation in the days before a formal hearing took place.

Like the conflict over staff assuming they could occupy office buildings during times designated by protesters as periods of shutdown, the issue raised by the incident was deeply enfolded into meanings of taking the decolonial project beyond cosmetic change. On the one hand were the orderly rules and procedures for dealing with allegations of sexual assault and harassment, enshrined in various policies, and supposedly implemented by specially trained staff. The procedures spelled out protections for complainants, but stressed the rights of the accused to due process. In the view of protesters, the system was weighted heavily against complainants, and over the years there were many complaints where "due process" ended with alleged perpetrators being free to roam the campus, with all the dangers of traumatic encounters between themselves and complainants. There was, of course, also the possibility that those accused might reoffend. Worries about the way the system worked included burden of proof placed on the shoulders of victims, and methods of policing boundaries between complainants and alleged perpetrators before cases were heard.

There was an impulse among some in the protest movement to take the procedures around alleged sexual violence into their own hands by publishing testimonies on social media, about any incident in contention, and also deficits in the university's response through "due process" (Bennett, 2009). Ranged against this line of action were staff uniformly warned not to pre-empt or derail procedures in any way. The conflict that surfaced about sexual harassment and violence was deeply embedded in the decolonial project. At its centre was the image of colonial oppressors exploiting, neglecting or abusing the bodies of black women. The contestations around gender in the decolonial project will be explored further in Chapter 8.

The woman immediately responsible for the processes of reporting, counselling and making plans with faculty about the students' immediate academic trajectory following the storeroom incident felt overwhelmed and suddenly unsteady with procedures that were familiar and well worn. Fearing attack from both sides of the "due process" debate, she looked beyond her own immediate departmental circle for an authority to instruct her in an unambiguous way. Unfortunately, large institutions often excel at delivering mixed messages, and, to the extent that they compartmentalize, contradictions were inevitable. All this took place against a fierce rhetoric tearing at the edifice of the rules themselves. She began to doubt her own credibility, as well as the reliability of the institution in holding her through the growing storm. Students gathered in protest specifically about the storeroom incident, and for a time she was very directly under siege, with few allies on either side of the struggle. She was also encountering trauma triggered by the protests, the storeroom incident, and the talk circulating about many other incidents of sexual harassment and violence. That she remained open to hearing this many-sided story was greatly to her credit, and by her own account cost her dearly in terms of constant worry and inability to attend to work of her own.

At times during this period, the staff member described being strongly protective of all the students she taught, and angry with the "university" for their muddled assistance and apparent negligence of sexual violence on campus. On the other hand, she was angry about the extent to which the protest movement had disrupted the academic year, and burdened herself and her staff with the ruins of courses, some of which would probably never be completed. Her accounts of the dilemmas facing her had the character of describing something outside of herself. While there was something traumatized and shut down in her description, it also carried the kind of doubleness, the re-presenting perspectives from many sides that signalled a widening range of sight. As time passed, being blown to smithereens and falling forever gave way to a melancholic cohesion and an embrace of surrender to the power of events external to herself. She no longer accorded herself the authority to carry the mantle of institutional power, although she also did not abdicate from responsibility. It was a complex deferral of action, seeing a world made new. She used her doubleness of vision to craft startling juxtapositions, humorous contradictions, an ironic highlighter that both valued and played with her defrocked coloniality.

The following experience related to me in the course of the protests gave me further insight into the complexity of living in transitional zones between subjectivities. Immersed in thinking through the students' demands for a new way of being in her department, and as a broker between students and management, a woman on the academic staff described a structure within a structure within a section. While the outer rings had worked closely with the protesters' demands for curriculum change and a shift away from forms of teaching they felt were replicating old lines of power, an inner circle barricaded themselves away from such negotiation. The split between staff had led to conflict in meetings, and for some disengagement from both sides of the debate. Each side felt misidentified by the other, and suspicion infested attempts to plan ways to bring the academic year to completion. This staff member had sacrificed her own research projects in order to take on some of the duties of a colleague in a state of traumatic depletion. Her attempts to be a comfort to both students and staff traumatized by the protests seemed to have been regarded as either treacherous or a waste of time. In her experience, there was ruthlessness in the assault on the meaning of her efforts. At the same time, she was providing a holding space for students and staff needing to be heard and soothed. She was thinking of resigning, a statement in the moment of sacrifice, of being willing to be eaten, as Winnicott suggests in "The Depressive Position in Normal Development" (Winnicott, 2002, p. 276). This was a complex moment, for her signalling the doubleness of shifting consciousness. To resign would be an act of protest against a hierarchy she had felt was denigrating with respect to her scholarship. It felt like an act of immolation. She was double, coming forward in rage and fleeing in shame. She held all sides but became herself full of holes.

The rupture caused by shattering a habitual way of relating to objects – in their loved and hated hallucinatory appearance in internal worlds – affected both staff and students, leading to proliferations of objects bifurcated by splitting. As the masks began to slip for students protesting against their alienation from a campus imprinted with what they experienced as class and race privilege, there were moments of triumph, of commanding the abjection of former oppressors, and making imperious demands for a new regime. There were also many moments in which the lines of trauma caused by growing up in a historically oppressive society, and suffering under the weight of struggle to become materially and academically successful despite generations of discrimination and poverty, were by necessity expressed as a weeping into the cries of triumph. The two strands of the discourse were indissoluble, and indeed the triumph was itself traumatic, bringing in its wake the bundles of anxiety that blowing a world to smithereens must carry in its wake. Where students at times during the protests carried the day, occupying buildings, halting lectures, rallying large crowds to their cause, there was festivity and celebration, but also a spilling out of the accumulated trauma. Injustice done needed to be acknowledged publicly, with reparation offered, before a full working through of grief could begin. In the trauma testimonies, both public and private, that impelled the protest movement forward, individuals were both performing and experiencing black pain. The trauma of which they spoke was not a narrative separate from its endless internal repetition.

This was made more complicated by two factors. First, the way in which traumasong (McPhillips, 2017; Swartz, 2017) fuelled anger and mobilized solidarity within the protest movement tended to work against the unique quality of every person's traumatic experience, overriding in particular its complex relationship internally with rage, shame and guilt, the driving forces behind repetition and breakdown threatening always to recur.

Second, trauma testimony was received by management in ways that added to this misrecognition. There were public offers to all students of access to counselling, and promises of change to systems that had in general been experienced as alienating. Public trauma testimony given by individuals cannot be met, held and survived in ways that surrender to the possibility of repair through generalities. More intimate and trusting spaces would be essential for such a meeting. The traumasong of students as they allowed themselves to be seen brought with it the danger of pain being amplified in the way it lionized trauma as a category of psychological event without preserving the particularity of meaning for every person suffering. In this way, institutional recognition of a class of problems repeated the problem. Most significantly, in the act of ripping off a mask, refusing to be compliant to a colonial setting by hiding ongoing distress, students speaking of their trauma were confronted with another doubleness in the tension between public performance, wide but crude recognition, and a need to be recognized as suffering individuals by structures that had failed.

One example will illustrate. A black female student in a demanding postgraduate programme was asked to do a presentation to a number of her peers and teachers. The material to be delivered was complicated, and the subject matter touched directly on her life history. She received feedback from staff, all of whom she experienced as alienated from the decolonial struggle, that her presentation was academically inadequate. There were also comments made on her manner of delivery, which was described as "disengaged" and "flippant." Already struggling with her course of study, and resonating with the traumasong of the protests, the student became overwhelmed with shame (not being good enough for this elite university) and anger at being judged in ways that made her feel demeaned and powerless. She also felt cast back into a family history that had been marked by intergenerational trauma. After a weekend of lying in bed, she had taken a small number of sleeping pills to relieve herself of the burden of consciousness for some hours.

She had been active in the protest movement and had been able to put words to some of her own experiences of alienation on campus in various public meetings. At the same time, her relationship to her own family included strong expectations of compliance to their expectations of her, and a tendency to brush aside lifelong struggles with shame and anxiety. Multiple roles fractured her: she felt safe enough in protest circles, but was also reluctant to take a leading role in planning and organization. There was pressure on her from her parents to complete her degree. She felt hurt and misunderstood by academic staff, indelibly associated with the power to judge her as deficient. In this situation of being blown to pieces internally, mirrored in the campus smithereens, she sought help first from a foreign student from an African country with decolonial struggles long past. Perhaps this ally, not directly associated with either side of the protests, or subject to peculiarly South African trauma around ways of being interpellated into racial trauma, gave her a zone in which she was temporarily able to experience the pain of her situation, for a moment, as singular, hers alone. Over several weeks, she made tentative approaches to one member of staff with whom she had a relatively trusting connection, asking for advice and comfort. In doing this, she felt the danger of betrayal and betraying; far from surrendering to the space, she was able to use it only as a hypothesis of what help might be should it miraculously appear.

It was an in-between place, between family, staff and students. It was between campus violences, a violent inner world and not wanting to live, and between a ruthless demand to disrupt, coming from the protest movement, to interrupt courses, and a need to complete a degree.

In this section, I have described at some length ways in which I witnessed the impact on individual subjectivities of the protest movement. I see attention to this as critical to a mapping of a decolonial project that has lasting change to internal and often unconscious assumption of privilege as a central focus.

In a final example, I turn to the issue of my own subjectivity as a witness to the events described above. I would not have been a witness of any worth, or with any but the dimmest access to sight, had I not been undergoing my own process of being blown to pieces. This addresses one part of Jessica Benjamin's (2011) insistence on the complexity of both witnessing and building a third. The position of being a witness, often used in relation to courts or legal proceedings, suggests the act of seeing and vouching for the credibility of someone's account. In this role, witnesses may verify (I saw what you are describing and testify therefore to its truth claims). Witnessing might also mean resonating with an account, providing an experience of sharing a subjective field, and in this way helping those so witnessed not to feel alone. Sometimes witnessing suggests a triangle, a witness's eyes on the duelling pair. Invested in this might be the force of judgement and the privilege of not having to take sides; it might also be the repository of a shared moral third (Benjamin, 2017). Regardless of how the term is contextually situated, it implies multiplicity – seeing through the eyes of another, seeing two sides, considering competing truth-claims. All require deferring the imposition of a personal perspective on those of others, and a capacity to see oneself from the outside, as others might.

There were many moments in which the ongoing protests confronted me with a view of myself from the outside, as others saw me. The gift of doubleness this offered, painful and disorienting at the time, unanchored me from an identity I had in many ways taken for granted, and the rearrangement of internal furniture very directly created space for new experiences and new lines of narrative. One example will illustrate this.

The students had called for lectures to be cancelled until certain demands were met. Protesters, students and workers were marching down an avenue between university buildings, and on their way they entered each building they came to in order to make sure that no lectures were taking place. Where there were lectures, they asked the lecturer to stop and the audience to leave the lecture theatre. At this point, there was considerable support for the strategy, from the student body and some of the academic staff too. As the procession reached the building in which my faculty had its main offices, students found the main doors locked. Knowing that this might lead to an unnecessary confrontation, I slipped into the basement of the building, back up the inside stairwell, and unlocked the doors, which allowed the students into the lobby. They then made sure no lectures were being given and left. I stood on the front steps, and looked out over the crowd, filled with what I identified at the time as admiration for the discipline and vigour of this quest for transformation that I strongly supported the need for. Seeing me smile, two young women walking past said to each other, "Look at that woman smiling! This is all a joke to her. It's not a joke!"

I felt misrecognized. I wanted to run after the women, explain, find a way to put balm on this puncture in my self-esteem. I smarted and ruminated. And then much later I thought. Standing on the stairs, above the crowd. Watching, not marching. Smiling, not mirroring the anger and pain that was making its way along the avenue. Enacting my privilege. I conferred something, I bestowed pride as if I owned something. Not a joke indeed.

This example points to the ways in which my self, both conscious and unconscious, was brought into view. It also illustrates the ways in which I experienced my subjectivity constructing itself in relation to ways in which others constructed me. A fantasy about myself was opened to dismantling, bringing with it in the moment a sense of going to pieces and shame. In particular, a fantasy of myself as wanting to be helpful was exposed. To imagine oneself as "helpful" is in itself *unhelpful* in that it claims a privilege, a general gift of helpfulness to be bestowed with generosity. It signalled my wish to identify with those speaking rather than being allowed to listen.

The place of recognition in the colonial situation

In terms of recognition theory, to reach a place of mutual recognition, which asks for a new subjectivity, may mean periods during which the ruthlessness of the struggle denies the humanity of the other. For Winnicott, it is only after survival of ruthless attack that concern – the possibility of mutual recognition – makes its appearance (Winnicott, 1969). In Jessica Benjamin's influential elaboration of Winnicott's explication of the creation of externality through destruction and survival, the collision, the zestful demand, is the necessary precursor to the recognition of the other as "a centre of experience" (Benjamin, 1995, p. 70). It is the impact of one on another, and survival of that impact, that allows for reassurance that the other has an existence outside of projective fantasy. This, of course, describes the movement of object relating to object usage in infant development, but Benjamin has elaborated significantly on the narrowly focused developmental context that was Winnicott's point of departure to consider the repetitive dimensions of the collision in terms of a master/slave dynamic in situations of social and political conflict (Benjamin, 2017). In this body of work, she describes conflict, the splitting and projection that inserts and reinserts a wedge between polarized groups. She points to ways through its destructive effects by means of mutual recognition. It is a process that takes account of the two group subjectivities, each conferring "thingness," a dehumanized one-dimensionality on the other, and captured in the resonance of "only one can live" (Benjamin, 2017; Fanon, 1986, p. 218; Levi, 1988). It provides a solid basis on which intersubjective or relational interventions make a contribution to the understanding and resolution of social and political conflict. The trajectory, as described both in the Winnicott papers and by Benjamin, implies a developmental shift from "primitive" object relating (which negates the subjectivity of the other) to recognition, in which externality and the survival of two positions and subjectivities has been achieved.

The Winnicott and Benjamin accounts both place centrally the idea of collision of needs, their negation and negotiation, in a dynamic, as enabling the recognition by each side that both "can live." The negotiation is an exchange taking the players beyond either omnipotent control or folding into compliance that characterizes a master/slave dynamic. The collision therefore is regarded as potentially fruitful.

There is an important contrasting view, which dismantles fundamentally the basis for movement through collision to survival in Donna Orange's work that places "recognition as," reached through empathic immersion and mutual intersubjective vulnerability as the central element allowing change:

> Perhaps we should give up the search for the Hegelian self-conscious subject, with its implied demand for the other to re-cognize and create it. Instead, psychoanalysis, pursued in a non-authoritarian atmosphere of respectful dialogue, can make people more at home in their own experiential worlds. They thus become more able to participate in the dialogic processes of the larger human communities of which they can increasingly feel like members. The most important Gestalt-shift, or new "way of seeing," for many of our traumatized, humiliated, and degraded-feeling patients, can be the self-experience as a worthy participant in human conversation.
>
> (Orange, 2010b, p. 241)

The profound shift here is away from recognition of subjectivities as equivalent centres, towards providing the conditions under which there might be freedom of self-experience without impingement from or coercion by the other. It seeks, in Winnicott's words, a situation in which the good-enough environment mother (as distinct from the object mother, who in fantasy is being attacked) has the function of continuing "to be herself, to be empathic towards her infant, to be there to receive the spontaneous gesture, and to be pleased" (Winnicott, 1965, p. 76).

The difference between Jessica Benjamin's position and Donna Orange's could be viewed quite simply as straddling the gap between a model that prioritizes aggression and the theatre of conflict with the object mother, and one that prioritizes trauma, and looks to the environment mother to hold a space in time, be empathic and to receive the fullness of a self-experience, without negating or impinging. Pumla Gobodo-Madikizela's work provides an important commentary on what this fullness might be (Gobodo-Madikizela, 2003, 2008). Each position has radical implications for thinking about both development and ways of encountering the other. The one position privileges and expects mutual respect, to come out of emergent definition of selfhood through coming up against; the other, as Donna Orange summarizes in relation to the work of Emmanuel Levinas, unseats this privilege. She describes this in the following way:

> The face of the suffering other, he proclaimed, places an infinite and unfulfillable demand on me: You shall not kill; you shall not leave me to die alone. You are responsible for me. One's own subjectivity is a secondary result, what philosophers call an epiphenomenon, of responding to the other who, in his or her destitution, always transcends me. Levinas presents, I believe, a forceful challenge to the contemporary focus on the psychoanalyst's or therapist's subjectivity. "It's not about you," he might have said – except as you respond to or neglect the other.
>
> (Orange, 2010a, p. 11)

My intention here is not to debate the merits of these contrasting positions, but to consider their application to the work of psychiatrist and revolutionary psychoanalytic thinker Frantz Fanon, whose work is central to the decolonial movement in South Africa and elsewhere. The focus is on the subjective experience of change, the inner landscape of privilege and its abjection twin, and the place of recognition in the decolonial project.

Winnicott, Fanon and survival

The protests had material change in the university as their goal, but dismantling the experience of alienation, entailed in being forced into living as masked participant, was always a goal as well. Is material change an analogue for the internal changes critical to throwing off internal experience of being shackled to a colonial situation? Does one change as the other changes? The encounters I described above suggest four points: that turmoil in the outer landscape brings inner turmoil, to all concerned; that the nature of this turmoil might trigger deeper-seated, older layers of trauma; that for some, turmoil activates defensive hostility, while for others there is anxiety, dissociation, falling to pieces, and perhaps in time new ways of thinking; and finally, inner turmoil is no analogue of external change. Both are variable and have many strands. Moreover, I would suggest that an internal landscape shattered through the prospect of an outer reality being dismantled cannot be contained easily simply through the assurance that demands for material change are being met. The tsunami inside (Bromberg, 2008) has its own trajectory, and must be contained by resonance of thought and feeling. It needs also to be anchored to a narrative that describes inner rather than outer weather. While this might suggest a role for recognition, or recognition as, in this case of the dismantling of colonial privilege, the process also calls for counter-recognition.

The colonial situation sets up a master/slave dynamic in which the wretched are recognized as wretched; liberal iterations allow the privileged to mitigate wretchedness with certain constrained freedoms. Counter-recognition rejects altogether the need to be a part of this dynamic, regardless of its changing terms. This complicates the landscape of both ruthlessness and the arrival of ruth.

In this case study, I have described a sequence of events. First, there is a protest movement that organizes a ruthless attack on the paraphernalia of colonial privilege. Rituals, artworks, monuments fall.

Next, the class structure underlying privilege is brought sharply into view (Jansen, 2017). Under the spotlight is the situation of workers racially humiliated, and characterized as unprotected by the institution, and earning little to service the campus. Access to university education for those without wealth becomes a central issue for the protests, and the demand that university fees must fall is a rallying cry. All of this takes place amidst marches, rallies, closures and occupations of buildings. There are many practical, material changes that follow from the initial protest action. This leaves in its wake trauma and inner turmoil, and also the imperative to establish counter-recognition.

In *Black Skin, White Masks*, Fanon sets out the imperative to act, not react, to a master/slave dynamic: "For the French Negro the situation is unbearable. Unable ever to be sure whether the white man considers him consciousness in-itself-for-itself, he must forever absorb himself in uncovering resistance, opposition, challenge" (Fanon, 1986, p. 222). The unbearableness of being, even if the dismantling of colonial regimes has begun, is because an identity, based on misrecognition, has been *conferred*: "One day the White Master, *without conflict*, recognized the Negro slave. But the former slave wants *to make himself recognized*" (Fanon, 1986, p. 217).

On the one hand, there is a struggle, a collision, that both makes and demands a recognition: in Jessica Benjamin's terms, it might be a precursor to "both may live," in an assertion that "I too have a life and you do not have the privilege of conferring on it either its value or meaning." It is only after this assertion that a place of mutual recognition might be reached. For Donna Orange (2010b), the place of recognition as is reached through *undoing the act of sight* bestowed by the White Master, without full understanding. The question this raises is whether reaching this vulnerability of mutual recognition, or recognition as, can be found within the decolonial project, with its harbingers of unmantling, defacing, unsettling and calling attention, interrupting and being in every way ruthless. There is, too, the critical issue of the terms of recognition, and whether, in a colonial situation undergoing displacement, it has a role to play at all in reaching for ruth.

Fanon's essays, particularly those on violence and its place in the necessary rupture with the white privilege embedded in colonial and postcolonial situations, place a radical shift in consciousness at the centre of revolutionary action:

> If, in fact, my life is worth as much as the colonist's, his look can no longer strike fear into me or nail me to the spot and his voice can no longer petrify me. I am no longer uneasy in his presence. In reality, to hell with him. Not only does his presence no longer bother me, but I am already preparing to waylay him in such a way that soon he will have no other solution but to flee.
> (Fanon, 2004, p. 37)

This is war with a persecutory object, the object mother, and a "clear image . . . within the grasp and imagination of every colonized subject . . . to blow the colonial world to smithereens" (Fanon, 2004, p. 37). Then: "I find myself suddenly in the world and I recognize that I have one right alone: That of demanding human behavior from the other. One duty alone: That of not renouncing my freedom through my choices" (Fanon, 1986, p. 229). And: "Yes to life. Yes to love. Yes to generosity" (Fanon, 1986, p. 222).

For Winnicott, the "yes to life" of which Fanon writes is the expression of the true self, the spontaneous gesture. It is not self-conscious, but must be received if it is not to be translated into false consciousness or compliance. It is zest always in the making and seeking to be seen. Its demand for recognition is ruthless and entails a necessary displacement of the other's gesture in the inner world. Through this is displaced the rule of the other inwardly, and it establishes the boundary between inner and outer, without which reality is a thing, a dead letter untouchable by imagination, severed from creativity, unenlivened by the shimmer of desire. To read this in terms of Fanon's call for action: here, the spontaneous gesture is the image of blowing the colonizers "to smithereens." Ruthlessness allows the shift to occur (see Benjamin, 1995; Villet, 2011). It also establishes ruth, the "yes to love, yes to generosity." It is not mutual recognition, but counter-recognition, a defiance of the need to be recognized. The decolonial situation radically displaces the players in the master/slave dynamic, demanding, on the one hand, reparation for damage done (*as if that were possible*), and at the same time rejecting the dynamic link itself.

Fanon is talking about a manifesto for action through which disalienation might occur. Instead of being "drowned in contingency" (in which self can only be experienced in the terms set out by the other), "invincible dissolution" is needed (Fanon, 1986, p. 218), one consciousness shifting to another. This is the process through which destruction might lead to a reconstitution, or, in Winnicott's terms, dissolution of a world made precarious by object relating, becoming a new consciousness in which object usage "puts the brakes on" fantasy (Winnicott, 1969). It can be assumed in this model that the interlocutors on both sides of the conflict move from "primitive" defense to the "maturity" of accessing a reality no longer split into good and bad, or riven with persecutory anxiety. The spontaneous (and rageful) gesture is necessary; it must be received, and the rupture implies loss and trauma. The suffering other is the infinite demand, before, during and after the gesture, the disruption. This is not a movement simply from "primitive" to "mature"; on the contrary, there is a constant oscillation between object relating and object usage, between ruthlessness and its necessary single-mindedness and experience of the full signification of suffering consciousness within.

The difficulty in translating this into Fanon's demand for action is that he is talking about, on the one side, an expansive and colonizing subjectivity that shapes inner and outer worlds, and, on the other side, a subjectivity doubled, and experiencing colonization alongside an apprehension of what it means to be human. It is the doubling of consciousness that calls for a doubleness in resolution, one part recognition of trauma, and one counter-recognition, a refusal to be recognized through the eyes of the colonizer.

One strand to the decolonial struggle is embedded in the necessary dissolution of privilege, the blowing to smithereens. The level of trauma implied for both parties to the collision is catastrophic; opportunities for repetition of past wounds proliferate; enactments abound. Here, suffering is the unfillable, infinite demand. The "secondary result," a reworked, renewed subjectivity, then creates possibility of many other layers of recognition. This points both towards Donna Orange's "recognition as," and the possibility of recognition through equivalent subjective centres.

The argument needs to be taken one step further. In the decolonial struggle, what is to be recognized, and by whom? There is an uneven landscape of privilege here. "Standing" is itself contested. For the colonized, recognition conferred by the colonizers is always doomed to be a form of patronage. Fanon is clear that "human behaviour," the "I am" of true selfhood free from contingency, is needed, but the "I am" of colonizers, enmired in centuries of privilege, is always less than human, because it simply reasserts the privilege of being, without first giving it up. Moreover, to weigh the suffering of the colonized in scales that attempt to incorporate colonizer suffering as part of the dynamic is deeply problematic. For colonizers to abdicate, making a silent retreat to the sidelines also seems like no solution: being left to blow an absence to smithereens repeats another act of privilege, rehearses old violences of relocation and absence by colonizers, the gift of being mobile. Colonizers must be there to be defaced and to create for themselves the "I am" that might stand steadily in a landscape reinvented, and shaped by entirely different lines of privilege.

The endless drift, precipitous worries and black holes of the inner-world anxieties is contingent on the capacity of the real world to reassure. There is paradox in the fact that the capacity to be alone, the "I am," depends on the holding environment. This is less about a "standing" in a landscape than the landscape itself remaining steady. In decolonization, this cannot be assumed: territories themselves change hands, institutions reshape, constitutions are reworked, the land moves under foot.

The "primitive edge" of protest

It is no surprise that descriptions of protest action in both social media and political or academic discussions draw attention to its challenge to "due process," to law and order, routine and rationality. This is unsurprising because protest action has disruption as a goal; it comes into being as a challenge to the naturalized order of things. The bundle of words that surface and resurface around protests concern not only rupture – the tearing of a social fabric – but also the designation of rallying crowds as potentially violent "mobs," susceptible to irrationality. This is "the primitive edge" (Ogden, 1989), and while it might be a way to understand some parts of protest action, it carries with it a logic that is easily imported into theorizing solutions to conflict. In this logic, those on opposing sides of impassioned conflict are locked defensively into "primitive" defences such as projection and splitting. This suggests that the way forward might be mapped in terms of a movement away from childish demand and into adult negotiation. Through this line of argument, there is also a connection to "true" or "primary" states of being. In this trope, infantile mental states are a window into the savage joys and terrors of the unconscious, before it is covered over by a veneer of adaptation to the demands of polite society. This section seeks to complicate this logic. There are two parts to the argument. In Winnicott's explication the movement from object relating to object usage is a developmental achievement. The other is about the meaning of holding, "recognizing as" and witnessing, each of which has the capacity to insert privileged maturity (at least in relation to object usage) into a dynamic that positions "primitive" emotional states as needing to be contained.

I have suggested that the process of changing subjectivities through collision in protest movements is necessarily traumatic. Before there can be new wholes, there are shatterings, splitting and dissociation, projection and doubling up in pain and contradiction. The catastrophe of seeking to be found and finding oneself lost, bearing misrecognition, colliding, falling forever instead of being caught, are all agonies, as Winnicott describes in "Fear of Breakdown" (Winnicott, 1989). It is, however, fundamentally problematic to cast a demand for freedom from contingency into the terms of a developmental trajectory that maps the struggle as a movement from relentless demand to "mature" ambivalence and respectful consideration of multiple points of view. In the decolonial situation, there are indeed multiple points of view to be recognized, at different points in the struggle, but this is not necessarily best cast as a developmental trajectory, taking opponents from "primitive" conflict to "mature" negotiation. The decolonial project imagines rehumanizing those colonized in their own terms; it therefore has far more than ruthless attack of colonizers at stake, in seeking terms for subjective survival outside of a colonial dynamic.

Further, a logic that places tumultuous conflict in the process of decolonizing as emotionally "primitive" fundamentally reiterates a traumatic history of colonial regimes, identifying themselves as "civilized," being attacked by those resisting being colonized (Brickman, 2003; Swartz, 2015). It is precisely these terms of engagement that decoloniality rejects.

There are three further points to be made in relation to the "primitive" in a protest movement seeking to humanize. First, it is a term used to describe mental states associated with infancy, despite ongoing work demonstrating the sophistication of babies' adaptation to complex caregiving surrounds (Beebe and Lachmann, 2013). It is also used to apply to adults in regression, or under the sway of tumult, fragmentation or disorder (Ogden, 1989; Samuels, 2015; Winnicott, 2002). All these forms of marking tumultuous emotional states on a continuum of maturity risks rehearsing colonial insistence on a single form of "civilized" affect regulation, and is always in danger of describing the affective displays inflected by cultures alien to that of colonizers as disorderly and a threat.

Second, groups (in this case, protest movements) have long been thought of as holding collectively "primitive" thought processes and defences. In Freud's words, "A group is impulsive, changeable and irritable. It is led almost exclusively by the unconscious" (Freud, 1921, p. 81). In this account, Freud was strongly influenced by the French sociologist Le Bon, in whose view "An individual in a crowd is a grain of sand amid other grains of sand, which the wind stirs up at will" (Le Bon, 1895/1960, p. 33). We would not have parties if we were unaffected by groups, if we did get "taken out of ourselves," not relish the slightly wild conversations, the flirting and dips into emotional intensity and disinhibition that our everyday routines tend to disallow. We go to football stadia to get "carried away" by the crowd's support for "our" team. Speeches are made to get the rush of a crowd's approbation. And protest movements draw their oxygen from chanting, roaring, dancing, waving, exhilarated, angry, hopeful groups, which certainly put aside reflection briefly for the headier atmosphere of urgent action. However, to impute "mindlessness" or "primitive" emotional states to groups is problematic in a number of ways. Most importantly, it provides a ready excuse to undermine demands made by impassioned crowds as "irrational," and therefore unworthy of attention. It presupposes a model in which individual mindedness is erased by collective mindlessness. The idea that groups might function as one organism has been ratified by systems theory, which assumes their tendency to be "creative, resourceful, and whole" (Page, 2003). Recent work on perverse systems suggests that through the constitution of roles, groups might become self-defeating, neglectful or sadistic, and be creative, resourceful and whole, but far from wholesome (Chapman and Long, 2009; Long, 2002, 2009).

Both these formulations, however, depend on a model of group mindedness that erases individuals' thinking. Bion's influential account includes his insistence that understanding a group's emotional life "is only comprehensible in terms of psychotic mechanisms," and that while the working group is rational, basic assumptions, held beyond working group consciousness, are always pre-symbolic, with no conception of either time or the possibility of development (Bion, 1952 p. 247; see also Samuels, 2015). This denies strategy and the ways in which crowd leaders and monitors protect, empower and achieve significant victories over opposing groups. These are points underscored by Mitscherlich (1969) in relation to Latin American political protests, and tellingly illustrated by Hollander (2014). And finally, it simply does not account for the variability of within-crowd behaviour, with the quiet and anxious shoulder to shoulder with the exuberant, the determined marching in step with the preoccupied or ambivalent, and so on. The complexity of group behaviour is therefore not reducible to either the "primitive" or to the assumption of "being of one mind"; neither is borne out by the evidence (Schweingruber and Wohlstein, 2005).

Third, the term "primitive" is invoked to describe the defenses of groups collected together not in space, but through an identity such as "middle class and white" or "Catholic and queer". Fakhry Davids, describing post-9/11 Islamophobia, says:

> Pervasive, primitive anxiety in the West, triggered by the bombings on that day, was managed by the deployment of a paranoid organisation in which the world of Islam is viewed as the enemy – the source of the threat to the West.
> (Davids, 2011, p. 63)

This is an example of a view that proposes projective mechanisms operating across an us/them divide, with those who belong under the umbrella of a particular social identity experiencing unwanted parts of themselves as belonging to those with social identities marked as different from their own. Defences of projection and splitting maintain internal cohesiveness, and foster prejudice, stereotyping, hatred and violence towards those who are transgressive or different. There is a significant literature on how psychoanalytic theory might both analyse and intervene with this difficult dynamic (see Altman, 2006; Benjamin,

1988, 2017; Corbett, 2001; Dalal, 2009; Dimen, 2013; Gobodo-Madikizela, 2015; Hadar, 2013; Samuels, 2015; Ullman, 2011). It has the merit of trying for even-handedness in locating the "primitive" as being characteristic of both warring parties. For the decolonial project, however, it forms yet another iteration of coloniality, taking the form of those with analytic skill labelling others as projecting (for example).

For all these reasons, it seems politically problematic to brand individuals in protest movements as "regressed" or in thrall to the "primitive." I suggest that it is also inaccurate in terms of relational theory, in two ways: it denies the legitimacy, in an adult or "mature" emotional economy, of expressing rage, frustration or terror, and it carries the danger of muddling analytically an internal landscape with protest action in the outer world. The ruthlessness, agonies and unconscious fantasies of inner worlds of object relating eddy into affective expression during protests, but protests are not unmediated rampages of unconscious desires synchronized across individuals fused by membership of a group.

Discussion of the penetration of coloniality with the "primitive" must include some thought about the role of witnessing in the decolonial project. There is a colonial model for witnessing in the figure of the anthropologist, contemporaneous with the birth of psychoanalysis, writing ethnographies of "savage" tribes. This is a position deeply embedded in privilege. There are, of course, many other forms of witnessing: inserting oneself as scribe within a protest movement might be one; watching for and reporting incidents of abuse or brutality is another; and a third is a form of engaged witnessing in which the aim is to listen with care and compassion to a variety of experiences as they unfold during times of crisis. "Recognition as" depends on this kind of witnessing, and critically is predicated on receiving an invitation to a conversation; there can be no respectful or humanizing exchange in its absence. To be a witness to traumasong involves being seen by those sharing their experience as being able to receive it fully, with no pre-judgement or self-promoting motive. In terms of decoloniality, there is necessarily vigilance about witnesses inserting themselves into conflict as holders of reflectiveness, expert knowledge or maturity; it is exactly for these reasons that taking up a witnessing role of any kind demands a surrender of a personal stake. The "I am" of witnessing is one of surrender, but also of maintaining the capacity for ongoing thought. Both standing and privilege, conferred by the role of being witness, are always subject to renegotiation.

Seeing double and living through

The argument I have set out in this chapter has a focus on conflict, and the ways in which this might lead to the rearrangement of subjective and intersubjective worlds. What I have described has sometimes involved conflict between groups, but I have also suggested that collisions may include coming up against institutional structures, procedures and protocols, and even the ways buildings command space. I have suggested further that collisions are productive of psychological trauma, and also draw antagonists in to circumstances that make the repetition of earlier layers of trauma more likely. Finally, I have suggested that shifts in alienated or dissociated states that may be argued to characterize colonial subjectivity might require that those who have been protected by privilege enter a period of doubleness, of seeing themselves from the outside. Those blowing the colonial world to smithereens have trauma too, of past pain and present ruthlessness, an internal burden until survival is securely lived into being.

The shift in consciousness required by shedding coloniality as a state of mind has counter-recognition as the place in which a platform of equality and respect might be built. As Fanon argues, and the South African universities' experience confirms, recognition cannot be conferred. Paradoxically, while mutual recognition is a part of confirming subjective independence, and this implies a comparison between two subjectivities, the negotiation simultaneously implies an assertion of "being in itself," careless of the other, a ruthless demand to be taken in as separate. In the case of the South African universities' protests by students, the contradiction in this is illustrated celebratory sloughing off of a mantle of oppression previously endured, and an ongoing wish that this be witnessed and recognized by those oppressors. At times, the dynamic rehearsed itself as a powerful complementarity. As Jansen observes, there were times when "only one voice is allowed to speak, and that is the loud, angry, and collective voice of the hostile disruptor bringing a grievance into a public space" (Jansen, 2017, p. 128). Periods of what Jansen calls "unreason" sometimes silenced debate, but nonetheless these periods were sufficiently ruthless to rupture habits of consciousness malformed by colonialism.

Jansen's use of the word "unreason" does, however, need some thought. My argument suggests that rupture through collision, essentially an affective experience, is a route through alienation because it brings with it an imperative to navigate unsettling internal states. The turmoil lies in the failure of both habitual structures of thought ("reason") and old lines of affect regulation that embody unconscious experience (Knoblauch, 2017). It is a profound simplification to characterize such moments of heightened affect as "unreason" or an expression of the "primitive" needing "maturity" or "rationality," ego or superego, to corral its energy. Rather, situations allowing for emotional fluidity (Knoblauch, 2017) provide the necessary conditions for new states to emerge; reason will later organize these into narrative representation. As Knoblauch (2017, p. 306) suggests, "we can surrender to the possibilities for growth, recognition, and liberation that dysregulated emotional moments make possible, for breakthroughs made possible by breakdowns or breakups." Further:

> Experiences of thresholds constitute tensions of uncertainty and thick complexity. Much of analytic work consists of developing capacities to navigate and/or inhabit such emotional tensions for the new possibilities that can emerge rather than a collapse into old and inadequate categories of thought or strategies for action.
>
> (Knoblauch, 2017, p. 293)

It is fitting that this chapter ends by returning to the complexity that the project of decolonizing the mind requires. While protests provide moments of heightened affect that usher in new experience and lay the foundation for consolidating new and more stable states of consciousness in those able to bear the terrors of uncertainty, they also herald for those vulnerable to fragmentation an escalation of defensive rigidity. Moreover, as Knoblauch rightly emphasizes, surfing fluidity demands a widening of awareness and an ability to tolerate conscious perception of being deeply unsettled. Finally, in interactions between groups, exchange of shared moments of affective vulnerability remain volatile, and potentially traumatizing for some. Narrative structuring of any kind is both containing and distorting, translating the complexity of mutual affective readings to the clumsy obscurity of words. It is here perhaps that repetition – not of old coercive forms, but of newly established ones, to be lived in and worn through many reiterations, with small incremental adjustments as time goes by – is the survival and repair after rupture with the past has opened caves of space within.

Note

1 Throughout this chapter, I have preserved the anonymity of the individuals and departments I describe.

A short version of the central argument in this chapter will appear in an article entitled 'Counter Recognition in Decolonial Struggle' in Psychoanalytic Dialogues, 2018.

References

Altman, N. (2006). Whiteness. *Psychoanalytic Quarterly*, *75*(1), 45–72.

Beebe, B. and Lachmann, F. M. (2013). *Infant research and adult treatment: Co-constructing interactions*. Routledge.

Benjamin, J. (1988). *The bonds of love*. Pantheon.

Benjamin, J. (1995). *Like subjects, love objects: Essays on recognition and sexual difference*. Yale University Press.

Benjamin, J. (2011). Acknowledgment of collective trauma in light of dissociation and dehumanization. *Psychoanalytic Perspectives*, *8*(2), 207–214.

Benjamin, J. (2017). *Beyond doer and done to: Recognition theory, intersubjectivity and the third*. Routledge.

Bennett, J. (2009). Policies and sexual harassment in higher education: Two steps forward and three steps somewhere else. *Agenda*, *23*(80), 7–21.

Bion, W. R. (1952). Group dynamics: a re-view. *The International Journal of Psycho-Analysis*, *33*, 235–247.

Bosch, T. (2017). Twitter activism and youth in South Africa: The case of #RhodesMustFall. *Information, Communication & Society*, *20*, 221–232.

Brickman, C. (2003). *Aboriginal populations in the mind: Race and primitivity in psychoanalysis*. Columbia University Press.

Bromberg, P. M. (2008). Shrinking the tsunami: Affect regulation, dissociation, and the shadow of the flood. *Contemporary Psychoanalysis*, *44*(3), 329–350.

Chapman, J. and Long, S. (2009). Role contamination: Is the poison in the person or the bottle? *Socio-Analysis*, *11*, 53–66.

Corbett, K. (2001). More life: Centrality and marginality in human development. *Psychoanalytic Dialogues, 11*(3), 313–335.
Dalal, F. (2009). The paradox of belonging. *Psychoanalysis, Culture & Society, 14*(1), 74–81.
Davids, F. (2011). *Internal racism: A psychoanalytic approach to race and difference.* Palgrave Macmillan.
Dimen, M. (2013). *Sexuality, intimacy, power* (Vol. 22). Routledge.
DuBois, W. E. B. (1989). *The souls of black folk.* Bantam.
Fanon, F. (1986). *Black skin, white masks.* Pluto Press.
Fanon, F. (2004). *The wretched of the earth.* Grove Press.
Freud, S. (1921). Group psychology and the analysis of the ego. *The standard edition of the complete psychological works of Sigmund Freud, Volume XVIII (1920–1922): Beyond the pleasure principle, group psychology and other works* (pp. 65–144). Hogarth Press.
Gobodo-Madikizela, P. (2003). *A human being died that night: A South African story of forgiveness.* Houghton Mifflin.
Gobodo-Madikizela, P. (2008). Trauma, forgiveness and the witnessing dance: Making public spaces intimate. *Journal of Analytical Psychology, 53*(2), 169–188.
Gobodo-Madikizela, P. (2015). Psychological repair: The intersubjective dialogue of remorse and forgiveness in the aftermath of gross human rights violations. *Journal of the American Psychoanalytic Association, 63*(6), 1085–1123.
Hadar, U. (2013). *Psychoanalysis and social involvement: Interpretation and action.* Springer.
Hartman, S. (2005). Class unconscious: From dialectical materialism to relational material. *Psychoanalysis, Culture & Society, 10*(2), 121–137.
Hollander, N. C. (2014). *Uprooted minds: Surviving the politics of terror in the Americas.* Routledge.
Jansen, J. (2017). *As by fire: the end of the South African university.* Tafelberg.
Knoblauch, S. H. (2017). The fluidity of emotions and clinical vulnerability: A field of rhythmic tensions. *Psychoanalytic Perspectives, 14*(3), 283–308.
Le Bon, G. (1895/1960). *The crowd.* Viking.
Levi, P. (1988). *The drowned and the saved*, trans. R. Rosenthal. Summit Books.
Long, S. (2002). Organisational destructivity and the perverse state-of-mind. *Organisational and Social Dynamics, 2*(2), 179–207.
Long, S. (2009). Sad, mad or bad: What approaches should we take to organisational states-of-mind? *Psychoanalytic Studies of Organizations: Contributions from the International Society for the Psychoanalytic Study of Organizations (ISPSO)*, 241–260.
Long, W. (2017a). Essence or experience? A new direction for African psychology. *Theory & Psychology, 27*(3), 293–312.
Long, W. (2017b). Alienation: A new orienting principle for psychotherapists in South Africa. *Psychoanalytic Psychotherapy in South Africa, 25*, 67–90.
Long, W. (2018). Decolonising higher education: Postcolonial theory and the invisible hand of student politics. *New Agenda: South African Journal of Social and Economic Policy, 69*, 20–25.
Maldonado-Torres, N. (2016). *Outline of ten theses on coloniality and decoloniality.* Fondation Frantz Fanon.
Mamdani, M. (2018). *The African university.* Retrieved 18 July 2018, from www.lrb.co.uk/v40/n14/mahmood-mamdani/the-african-university.

McPhillips, K. (2017). "Unbearable knowledge": Managing cultural trauma at the Royal Commission. *Psychoanalytic Dialogues*, *27*(2), 130–146.

Mignolo, W. (2011). Epistemic disobedience and the decolonial option: A manifesto. *Transmodernity: Journal of Peripheral Cultural Production of the Luso-Hispanic World*, *1*(2), 44–66.

Mitscherlich, A. (1969). Introduction to panel on protest and revolution. *The International Journal of Psycho-Analysis*, *50*, 103–108.

Nyamnjoh, F. (2016). *#RhodesMustFall: Nibbling at resilient colonialism in South Africa*. Langaa.

Ogden, T. H. (1989). *The primitive edge of experience*. Karnac.

Orange, D. M. (2010a). *Thinking for clinicians: Philosophical resources for contemporary psychoanalysis and the humanistic psychotherapies*. Routledge.

Orange, D. M. (2010b). Recognition as: Intersubjective vulnerability in the psychoanalytic dialogue. *International Journal of Psychoanalytic Self Psychology*, *5*(3), 227–243.

Page, L. J. (2003). Adler and the profession of coaching. *Journal of Individual Psychology*, *59*(1), 86–94.

Samuels, A. (2015). *The political psyche*. Routledge.

Schweingruber, D. and Wohlstein, R. T. (2005). The madding crowd goes to school: Myths about crowds in introductory sociology textbooks. *Teaching Sociology*, *33*(2), 136–153.

Swartz, S. (2015). *Homeless wanderers: Movement and mental illness in the Cape Colony in the nineteenth century*. UCT Press.

Swartz, S. (2017). Collectively speaking: The many meanings of naming and sharing group trauma. *Psychoanalytic Dialogues*, *27*(2), 156–163.

Ullman, C. (2011). Between denial and witnessing: Psychoanalysis and clinical practice in the Israeli context. *Psychoanalytic Perspectives*, *8*(2), 179–200.

Villet, C. (2011). Fanon and recognition in the colonial context. *The Journal of Pan African Studies*, *4*(7), 39–51.

Winnicott, D. W. (1965). *The maturational processes and the facilitating environment: Studies in the theory of emotional development*. Karnac.

Winnicott, D. W. (1969). The use of an object. *The International Journal of Psycho-Analysis*, *50*, 711–716.

Winnicott, D. W. (1989). *Psycho-analytic explorations*. Harvard University Press.

Winnicott, D. W. (2002). *Through paediatrics to psychoanalysis: Collected papers*. Karnac.

Chapter 6

Rhodes, falling

Nestled against the grandeur of Table Mountain, and overlooking the sprawl of a divided Cape Town, a city part affluent, attractive to tourists from all over the world, but sheltering also communities ravaged by poverty, is the University of Cape Town.[1] As described in earlier chapters, it is a university with a long history, a tradition of scholarly productiveness, and visibility on the international stage (Swartz, 2016). The upper campus looks down, across the peninsula, a panoptical gaze, one that has many times been characterized as removed from the brutal reality of poor communities, the grime of shacks and smoke. This position – often described with one single word, elitist – has reverberated through generations of struggle. It is a liberal institution, committed to what Maldonado-Torres refers to as "liberal temporality," prioritizing order over change (Maldonado-Torres, 2016, p. 4). As a part of this liberalism, it has a track record of activism, opposition to anti-democratic political movements, and a vocal anti-apartheid movement that included both faculty and students through the 1970s and 1980s. There have also been inevitable moments of collusion, a turning away of scholarly faces away from the suffering clearly visible from the view from the hill. As a liberal institution, there was always belief in debate, in individual freedoms, in human rights, but the institution remained vulnerable to the charge of failing to rise to the challenge of decolonizing itself from a past saturated in white privilege.

Here was the landscape taken for granted by those who felt they "belonged" in the university community. It was shot through with access to privilege and property and with choice about trajectories of movement, partly because of its lordly position on the mountain flanks, with only the relatively wealthy living within easy walking distance from its campus. At every turn, it faced those who interacted with it with "prominence": "a projecting feature of the landscape or a protuberance on a part of the body" (*Oxford English Dictionary*). As the university "rose" up the ranks of world rankings, it became more "visible." It seemed unable to shake off the mantle thrown over its endeavours by ivy-covered buildings in the Oxbridge mould, pride in traditions, and a relatively unthinking set of assumptions about what universities do, what they create and how they should relate to the communities they serve. Most of all, the scholarly community was slow to deconstruct what it means to look north, from a promontory, to the United

Kingdom and the United States, for sanction and status, instead to the knowledges and wisdom of the African continent (Mamdani, 2018). "We" wanted to be part of a mobile but connected international community, one centred in the north. The idea of radically destabilizing that hub-and-periphery status quo was barely on the agenda.

What would it mean for the University of Cape Town to look inward first, and then to its own home, Africa, for its values, traditions and future planning? What does it mean to confront the fact that there is no "we," was no "we," will be no "we" until a way is found to share a common subjectivity?

Before 2015, persistent but often isolated voices raised these questions (for example, Barnes and Mama, 2007; Kamola, 2011, 2015; Mamdani, 1998; Ntsebeza, 2014), and to give the university's management its due, they were recorded as important debates in a variety of strategic plans and pledges, underpinned always by the liberal humanism that infused all its discourse, and committed it to the paradox of liberal movements everywhere: of self-preservation, on the one hand, and responsiveness to injustice and the urgent need to look into the face of those alienated, on the other (Orange, 2011). The rupture of 2015 entailed coming to terms with a colonial past, one preserved and defended for more than a century (Nyamnjoh, 2016).

This chapter will describe the rupture of 2015 and 2016 at the University of Cape Town, and the place of art and space at its centre. It was an impinging environment, in spaces experienced as still colonial in their effects. The relationship of art to these spaces, and the complex meaning of the defiant spontaneous gesture, the ruthless insistence on refusing compliance in relation to expression of the true self, will map the path through this colonial space.

I will describe the ways in which works of art become transitional objects, crafting the potential space within which new spontaneous gestures might arise. I will also suggest that works of art, in providing a transitional space between apparently objective representation of reality and subjective meanings, have an important role to play in the process of confounding alienation, disrupting compliance, and healing fractures between what is false and what is true. As Maldonado-Torres suggests, "in decolonial artistic creation, the embodied subject emerges as someone who can not only reflect about but also mould, shape, and reshape subjectivity, space and time" (Maldonado-Torres, 2016, p. 27).

Before the #RhodesMustFall protests, the university campus was adorned in various ways, partly in the statue-and-portrait style that celebrates and memorializes a particular kind of leadership, one that "institutes" and preserves a historical narrative. There were also original paintings large and small, sculptures and carefully curated exhibitions of artefacts with historical significance. Some of the adornments and works of art were compliant with the university's self-proclaimed identity; others were akin to dreams, the ruthless expression of a vision, an unconscious life, true selfness, disruptive in their encoded expression of the artists' and institution's unconscious life. Some of these expressions caught dreams that sought a rupture with the placidity of committee rooms and meeting halls. Others brought to some eyes, mine included, painful awareness of a placidity embraced, in enacting the right to comment on Otherness from a distance underwritten by privilege.

In the protests of 2015, it was the adornments transparently celebrating both tradition and colonialism that became a major focus of attention. This included, in particular, the statue of Cecil John Rhodes, and portraits of mainly white and male university luminaries. My argument in this chapter will be that their dismantling created potential space within which a new institution was beginning to be dreamed. The acts of dismantling became pieces of performance art, creating in their ruthless destruction a new landscape, the contours of which allowed a new identity to emerge.

In "Psycho-Analysis and the Sense of Guilt," Winnicott comments on the artist's ability to create without compliance to society, that is distinct from "guilt-driven labour" (Winnicott, 1965, p. 26). The links between spontaneity, an expression of a vision, the production of a work of art, and imperiousness to ways in which it might be received are embedded in notions of creativity and originality being at root the same thing. In charging the university's adornments with complicity in colonialism, protesters were mounting an attack on their originality. This becomes the critical pivot on which an unfolding dialogue between adornments, works of art, originality and complicity, and claim to voice began to be played out. The events described in the following sections trace the ruthlessness of the artist's gesture in the protests, and the expression of a rebellious vision counter to a historically sanctioned and compliant self. The tension between originality and compliance in an institution's representation of itself, and the paradoxes created by each, is a central scaffold.

Rhodes Must Fall

Here was the decisive moment. Chumani Maxwele, a politics postgraduate, assisted by comrades, threw human excrement at the statue of Cecil John Rhodes, hero and master-scavenger of colonial Africa. That there was a statue of Rhodes, gazing thoughtfully into the hinterland he planned to appropriate, had caused some disquiet, but until Chumani Maxwele's powerful performance of making a whole institution see the other Rhodes, a Rhodes with a legacy defiled by an oppressive and exploitative and dehumanizing colonial project, the effects of which has shaped us as a society, he had been lived with, partly seen, partly made invisible by the magic of dissociation, as we walked, rode or drove by (Bromberg, 2010). Regardless of what was "seen" or apprehended, moment by moment, the presence of the Rhodes statue, given its prominence, and the steep slope that fell away beneath his plinth conferred on him ownership of a landscape, a right to overbear.

After that, the dominoes toppled swiftly. There was debate, of course, about contextualizing the statue by having plaques noting his sullied history, or other works of art, talking back to him. But he proved to be a unifying symbol for the protest movement, in that sense paradoxically doing exactly what works of art must do. He impelled crowds to act, and he had to go. After weeks of this adornment being adorned with a variety of challenging counter-statements, such as garbage bags and toilet paper, he was boxed up, and eventually a crane swung him ingloriously on to the bed of a truck. He is now in storage, a room without a view.

Poo-throwing was an extraordinary piece of performance art. Encapsulated in it was not only a protest against Rhodes, and against the university as a colonial pile, preserving a history of white privilege, but also an enactment of thousands and thousands of poor households without water-borne sewerage, forced to use disposable toilets and live day in, day out with the stench of their own waste (Robins, 2014). The lines of battle were drawn.

Symbols are not the third

The contestation around the statue of Rhodes brought to the campus a moment of collective action, one that caught the imaginations of many, both nationally and internationally. Before it was removed, it was the site of rebellious counter-gesture, and there was vigorous disruption of his stony contemplation of the landscape: he was slapped and wrapped and labelled and smeared. A large crowd celebrated Rhodes being dethroned, a de-coronation taking place in a uniting, contagiously joyful atmosphere. Briefly, players on both sides of the drama elbowed their way forward to photograph the crane and the statue swaying its way on to the waiting transportation. It was a turning point, and marked a moment in which further transformation became inevitable. The empty plinth was very concretely a potential space, and this was used in a series of performance pieces, powerfully replacing Rhodes' panoptical gaze with living bodies demanding decolonization.

The de-coronation event constellated a third briefly, but just as the statue itself had divided, not provided, perspective, so too did its fall. On the one side was a group accusing management of collusion with the protests, buckling under pressure, and turning its back on the durability of history, whatever its evils. On the other, protesters claimed a victory over management, which foreclosed a mutual surrender into a space of negotiation. It was a powerful wave in which many swam as if "we" belonged. It had, however, none of the capaciousness implied by surrender to recognition, which requires an exchange, a letting in and embrace of separateness and difference, essential to thirdness (Benjamin, 2017, p. 23). The event was therefore a rehearsal, an opportunity for play and an immersion, a catharsis, necessary for the next step. The statue of Rhodes symbolized colonial violence. The action it precipitated, and the potential space it created in the total situation, signalled the possibility of a third to come, but this was not the moment in which surrender to something beyond complementarity could be achieved. Events surrounding the statue's removal were an extraordinary catalyst, but the campus was not done with a split dynamic. The falling of Rhodes as a powerful symbol quickly translated into "only a symbol," with the symbolic act needing to be followed up with substantive action.

Since Rhodes has fallen, the landscape is figuratively and literally transformed. The pace of transformation had left the campus all out of routine, worrying at times about going-on-being, a lack of continuity that had fundamental consequences for the integration of mind and psyche-soma, as Winnicott describes in "Mind and Its Relation to the Psyche-Soma" (Winnicott, 2002), discomforted and unsure, resonating each in our own way, and according to our histories with trauma uncovered. Stark lines of contestation had been drawn: on one side, management protecting (some would say being defensive about) both property and the usual administration of the academic project (now itself deeply contested), and, on the other, those calling for decolonization and free education, and an end to alienation in an environment experienced as elitist, the multiple microaggressions of racism, sexual harassment and trauma, and the burdens of generations of exclusion. Management was obligated to speak to rules and statutes and budgets. Across the chasm, black pain was voiced by deep and compelling voices, in rallies, classrooms, meetings and committees.

The fall of Rhodes' statue began a process of grappling with a place in which the ways that the university represented itself were now up for debate. No longer taken for granted was the logic of memorializing past wardens and vice chancellors in portraits hung in halls. Adornments of all kinds became contested, experienced by some as offensive, by others as representing a venerated tradition. The names of buildings tied to donor or scholarly contribution in the past became part of the change the community moved towards. While the buildings themselves remained obdurately seated and ivy-swathed, their ties to a colonial past swam uneasily into the foreground. There came an understanding that in this new landscape, there was a need for different heroes to venerate. For those who once claimed the privilege of belonging to this kind of an institution, who had felt "at home" in it, membership had to be earned, as it would not arrive unbidden. So, for some, there was a first experience of alienation, a mirror of all the painful acts of exclusion and alienation that have troubled and traumatized black staff and students for whole lifetimes (Swartz, 2007, 2012). This was only the beginning of the journey, part of which was to accept the principle that trauma unresolved is repeated, until a third might become possible (Aron, 2003; Benjamin, 2004; Black, 2003).

Shackville

I turn now to another decisive moment, again with a piece of performance art at its centre. Early in 2016, partly as a result of the turmoil of 2015, and examination rewrites, campus closures, and uncertainty about admission numbers, some newly registering students, mainly from black and underprivileged communities, found themselves on campus with no accommodation. The protest movement erected a shack between the oldest and most august residences on upper campus – the same ivy-covered halls that distinguished the campus as a whole as saturated in colonial history and modelled after Oxbridge forebears. The shack was quickly assembled, blocked traffic, and brought township poverty, lack of access to adequate housing and the shortfall in student accommodation into exquisite focus. It became an instant symbol for the social and economic disparities the university community had tended to ignore, defend against and dissociate from as it went about its daily business.

It was a telling performance, and the juxtaposition of the residences and shack inflamed a split so crudely emblazoned. The feelings it catalysed were too volatile to be held by either side, and in a night of violence, portraits and artworks, some representing white men and women who had presided over the residences, were put into a pile and were burnt. There were several incidents of arson and a petrol bomb was thrown through the vice chancellor's window. This was a point at which holding the split was an urgent need, but this proved to be an impossibility. Shackville was breathtakingly ruthless in its use of a boundaried space, and in its incisive commentary on homes, homing and being "at home." It was a vigorous attack on a stony mother; it was splendid in its assault on polite business as usual, canny in its use of symbol. The stone mother was called on to survive, not to retaliate, to listen and mould herself to what was being asked of her. Given the way big institutions operate, negotiations, meetings and conversations began, but were easily cast as slow or deceptive in their intent.

For a short time before the night of the burning, Shackville had created potential space, in the sense that it drew crowds, an enlivened audience, some critical but many curious and admiring, drawing breath from the fierce representation of disparity among students and staff between those with wealth and those with few resources. It was an enactment that marked the ongoing protests and the accommodation crisis as requiring immediate and sustained attention. As it ran its course, as it had to do, and there was a night of implosion, deep scars, polarized opinion, disciplinary action and also criminal charges were left behind. In the short term, potential space collapsed, dismantled along with the shack, to be replaced by a disquieting retreat into a space in which thinking itself had become difficult. A rupture had occurred, and this set the stage for the next piece of the process, and another reaching for survival beyond destruction, reassurance of the stability of object usage, and the possibility of the third.

Exhibiting #RMF

On the anniversary of the fall of the Rhodes statue, the RMF movement and the Centre for African Studies at UCT planned an exhibition, curated by Paul Weinberg, part photographic and part performative, of the events of 2015. This felt like a moment in which public memory might be materially constituted in order to become an object for reflection. An exhibition could be the occasion on which recognition and surrender to a new multiplicity in campus consciousness might be acknowledged, with photographs, videos, banners and artefacts from the beginning of the protests, many of which were shared extensively on social media at the time of their taking, contextualized and speaking beyond a simple moment-by-moment record to a collation, broader truths, an echo chamber of feeling and action. That this was the clear intention was captured in the exhibition's title, "Echoing Voices from Within: A Rhodes Must Fall Exhibition." The coloniality against which students were protesting was included in a "Contested Legacies" wall, which aimed to create a dialogue around the lasting material presence of colonial leadership on campus, and to open ways to speak back. In other words, the exhibition was to do what a work of art must do: speak in a way numinous enough to gather meaning, and be receptive to containing the contradictions brought by the audience's gaze.

Perhaps it was too soon. The exhibition was in the process of being officially opened when it had to be closed. The Trans Collective, a group of transgender, gender-nonconforming and intersex students and their allies, some naked, some in panties, all decorated with blood-red paint, entered, spoke, sprayed paint on the photographs, and lay on the floor, defying the audience to step over their naked bodies. They were protesting not only the selective memory crystallized in the exhibition, and their exclusion from representation, but also failure of consultation during the process of its curation. In their announcement, they made the following statement:

> This exhibition is taking place within a very current and still fluid political context. This exhibition is not a marker of a past historical event that is now over and that can be neatly portrayed behind glass in wooden frames. RMF is very current and the political action added to this exhibition by the Trans Collective is an important part of it and should be welcomed into it.

On the wall, a poster stated bluntly, "The Trans people who built RMF (Rhodes Must Fall) are not part of this exhibition."[2] Across a photograph of Chumani Maxwele throwing poo at Rhodes' statue, the word "rapist" abruptly challenged his leadership and his legitimacy in a movement proud to claim intersectionality as its guide to the transformation project. The disruption of the exhibition claimed that the RMF movement embodied:

> an outright refusal to acknowledge that the condition of being a womxn, queer, trans, disabled and so forth is not incidental to blackness but that these conditions are collateral to blackness. So suffocating is this that we have had to submarine from active membership. We refuse to avail our bodies and psyches for the violence that has infiltrated the decolonial project through patriarchy, cisnormativity, heteronormativity and the gender binary.
> (www.facebook.com/transuniversityforum/posts/1132209633512418)

Their message: this is not our memory. We refuse to be written out of a movement that we see as fundamentally patriarchal.

More dialogue was clearly needed. Would a more inclusive exhibition be an answer? And a question: in these contested spaces, who, or what, is memory or history? And without a stable narrative for either, how do we move towards object usage, as Winnicott described, or, in the language of Jessica Benjamin, recognition and surrender? Levels of contestation remained high, and the events surfaced suffering and trauma in individuals. Depression, anxiety and suicide tore at slim counselling resources. We were in many respects simply in need of holding, in that vulnerable and regressed space in which Winnicott, in "Metapsychological and Clinical Aspects of Regression," warns that it is case management, rather than analysis, that must be primary (Winnicott, 2002; see also Slochower, 2013).

Creating a third space: memory and art in question

In the aftermath of the initial Rhodes Must Fall mass action, which was quickly followed by demands that the university's workers be insourced, and that a halt be put to increases in university fees year on year, university management engaged extensively in negotiations with student and worker organizations, and in the course of this there were a series of tense confrontations between the vice chancellor, his senior management team and student activists. Often management stood accused of dealing in half-truths and pursuing oppressive means to maintain the status quo. Student activists were at times accused of negotiating in bad faith. Despite breakdowns in trust that felt irreparable at times, there was also dialogue uninterrupted: painful, stammering, but face-to-face. There have been substantial victories for the forces of change, but also survival and a holding of the frame by all sides.

What became clear during 2016 and 2017 was that the protests no longer contained a stable complementarity, a doer/done to dynamic in which heroes and villains are stably assigned, depending on the side to which each belonged. In its place were splinters, a fragmentation that publicly challenged the cohesion of the protest movement. And as the university's response to the protests unfolded, fractures could also be seen among staff bodies, some wishing that the stone mother would increase her stoniness, resist appeasement and become impervious to onslaught, while others demanded negotiation and compromise, admission of wrongdoing and wholesale change to usual ways of being.

Rhodes' statue, with its appropriative, colonizing gaze over the hinterland, aptly captured a colonial situation, not past, but concretely present. Removing it was emblematic of the undoing of colonial privilege. Importantly, the hero's status once conferred upon him by governments past was let go – publicly at least – with relative ease; it had almost no place in the debates surrounding the removal. The dismantling of the statue took with it the troubling symbol of a colonial past, and also served as a reminder that histories and the complicated truths of art are always contingent rather than timeless. More difficult was that the statue's removal failed to sustain potential space in which to represent history differently.

Shackville, with its juxtaposition of wealth and poverty, power and exclusion, was altogether more complicated than Rhodes falling. The spotlight was turned directly on to UCT's own heroes, wealth and history of privilege. What became clear was that transformation of the university would involve directly our own history, our own hierarchies and privilege, not only those of past regimes. As portraits were burnt, the fires etched two points with absolute clarity: that our institution needed to come to terms with its own history of exclusion and privilege, and this would entail necessary displacement of its symbols of that history, and that another history, one in the process of being articulated, was coming into being.

The RMF anniversary exhibition took this progression a step further. First, UCT's history was on trial, and its complicity with colonialism and apartheid exposed. And now the history of the student protests was itself being disrupted and rearranged. Memory itself was in disarray. History, too, is mutable, and this has important implications for the establishment of the third, which requires surrender from or to, a place from which to negotiate, a self that is able to represent, at least as a beginning, a continuity of being. Survival and everything that object usage promises by way of release from the coercions of omnipotent control that comes after destruction cannot be hurried, and is in any case continuously undone by internal attack. I am suggesting here that for an institution struggling with both memory and history, and also with existential threats brought about by difficult economic times, survival is not guaranteed, and this impacts on both potential space, and possibilities of building the third.

Repetition of trauma, ruthlessness and the idea of a university

There is much to be puzzled over and fretted about in this story. Time will help as we seek a version of events through the multiple and disputed versions that now confront us. There were, of course, contradictory truths, and into this volatile discursive space fell rumour and strategic disinformation, fuelled by a very active social media community. Despite a temporary muffling that felt dissociative, the university threw itself ruthlessly into something, a necessary dismantling of a thick set of assumptions and ways of being vital for the survival of the university as an object to be used (Winnicott, 1969, p. 713). It is to this that I now turn.

Concentration of wealth in the hands of a tiny minority of South Africa's population has perpetuated a situation in which the majority of its people live with poverty, poor access to healthcare and adequate education and housing, and high levels of unemployment. There are too many ways in which the traumatic effects of past inequalities reproduce, generation after generation, more than 100 years of oppression. The University of Cape Town campus, in remaining faithful to an idea of a "university," underpinned fundamentally by academic freedom, commitment to knowledge creation and a somewhat lofty separation from surrounding social and political contexts, has unthinkingly perpetuated this oppression in a number of ways. Forms of excellence, both in teaching and in research, have sought alignment with international benchmarks, and these inevitably foreclose on the salience of local knowledges. Its curricula, degree structures, rituals and hierarchies have allowed it to fit seamlessly into a much-prized list of world-ranked universities. This and a rich network of international links have brought both funding and security, but have also been faithful to a model of an institution with strong lines of continuity with both a colonial past and an affiliation with sister northern hemisphere universities. As Fanon notes in *The Wretched of the Earth*, universities have been responsible for a knowledge claim that "essential qualities remain eternal in spite of all the blunders men may make: the essential qualities of the West, of course" (Fanon, 2004, p. 11). The Rhodes Must Fall movement, in calling for decolonization of the university, was demanding that all this should change. In particular, it was insisting on a programme of radical transformation, one that would allow black South African students to feel a sense of both belonging to and ownership of the university as they studied.

This was not a modest demand, constituting nothing less than a rupture with the past. And here, the wisdom of psychoanalytic theory is helpful. It has been through the repetition of trauma, a playing out of a dynamic of oppression and alienation, and a visceral expression of the pain caused by each, that first brought the university to a standstill, and then moved all into furious thought, imagining the possibility of a different institution altogether. Critical to this change has been the way in which the comforts of belonging and identifying with the space have been abruptly removed from the privileged few.

At their best, universities create. They collate, discover, explore, debate. They allow students to play, and in playing to come to new minds. They are designed to be potential space, available to students as a source of recognition and independence. This entails destruction of previously unquestioned truth-claims and gatekeeping of access, and most significantly assumptions about what legitimately constitutes scholarship. In the spirit of play, students question and challenge; sometimes they prefer their own constructions to those of their elders. At the same time, this play is contained within limits that underwrite the university's survivability. There are curricula, assignment deadlines and in some disciplines an accumulative body of knowledge – elemental tables and laws of gravity – that bind student superheroes to earth. Universities are set up therefore to amplify the tension between rehearsal of what is already "common knowledge" and what is being excitedly created. Given this dynamic, it is no surprise that the way universities represent themselves might tread the path between veneration of elders and past scholarship, and the challenging production of the new. So, for example, in the performing and creative arts, there is immersion in centuries of music, writing, theatre and the arts, but always also the invitation to the original, in composition or interpretation.

What the Rhodes Must Fall movement called into question was fundamental to the disruption of the balance universities reproduce between rehearsal of the already known, so-called "fact" or "truth," and generation of the kinds of new knowledge that put the old at a slant, or tip it out altogether. Some of what had been venerated or taken for granted represented the colonial, and had to be uprooted and replaced with a new history, one that put in place a set of new "already knowns," originators of knowledge previously silenced or hidden by colonial regimes. This process is under way, but its instatement has brought a new volatility to the collision between creation and destruction through which object usage occurs. New elders, leaders, thinkers, now being memorialized by the institution for the first time, and recasting fundamentally its representation of itself as decolonial, African and belonging to Africa, will over time be established enough as iconic to survive the challenge to their legacy by the children; for now, veneration is both appropriate and an act of necessary restitution, involving idealization. But the flounder is in containing the dynamic that requires destruction to create, and to confirm survival, in the face of that idealization. As what can be taught and how it should be taught spawns new orthodoxies, there is a new wave of challenge to potential space, which was after all only ever an illusion.

Conclusion

I end this chapter with some thoughts on the conditions under which thirdness might be achieved in situations of ongoing conflict. The role of representation through art will be a specific focus.

The events described in the chapter provide a commentary on the mutability of connections between histories, memory and the representation of both in works of art. This instability and the space it creates is an opportunity for hearing, feeling and thinking anew, and in time more versions of history will come. During this tumultuous time, events constellated around artworks and performance pieces certainly opened debate, some on public platforms, some private. Hearts and minds have been changed, and the university community has been precipitated into a decisive rupture with old ways of being. There have been times when debates have foretold the coming of thirdness, but with a sense of fragility. And this is perhaps the point.

I have been wondering as time has passed what might help us to constitute a third space (for the complexity of this process, see Benjamin, 2016). We began with a statue, and it seems fitting that as we move forward we think about forms of art and representation, and whether it might provide a space to remember and reflect. The work of Kessi (2013) and Kessi and Cornell (2015) offers an instructive and encouraging example in this regard. Using Photovoice methodology, participants are asked to write stories about photographs they have taken. Exhibitions of these demonstrate with poetic and painful clarity subjective alienation of black students on a historically white campus, and the embodied nature of this alienation. The intimacy of the photographs and stories, their insistence on creating a reading of themselves, a standpoint that would say "I am" irrespective of the eye of a politically varied audience, was an act of generosity. The exhibitions spoke boldly, without equivocation; in this, paradoxically, they decolonized themselves from a space in which they spoke of the pain of being colonized. Intimacy and vulnerability contributed to an audience response resonant with emotion, and being dared to use this as potential space, a place in which embodied self-disclosure might be possible, and dreaming unformulated experience into a changed future might be possible (Ogden, 2014; Stern, 2013).

Notes

1 The events described in this chapter are richly illustrated by a series of photographs that appeared during the protests in social media. Interested readers may access them at www.facebook.com/RhodesMustFall/photos and www.facebook.com/transfeministcollective/photos.

2 Photographs of this extraordinary event, and the commentary, can be found at www.facebook.com/transfeministcollective/photos/pcb.1132209633512418/1132209240179124/?type=3&theater.

References

Aron, L. (2003). The paradoxical place of enactment in psychoanalysis: Introduction. *Psychoanalytic Dialogues*, *13*(5), 623–631.

Barnes, T. and Mama, A. (Eds.) (2007). *Rethinking universities II*. African Gender Institute.

Benjamin, J. (2004). Beyond doer and done to: An intersubjective view of thirdness. *The Psychoanalytic Quarterly*, *73*(1), 5–46.

Benjamin, J. (2016). Moving beyond violence: What we learn from two former combatants about the transition from aggression to recognition. In P. Gobodo-Madikizela (Ed.), *Breaking intergenerational cycles of repetition: A global dialogue on historical trauma and memory* (pp. 71–89). Barbara Budrich.

Benjamin, J. (2017). *Beyond doer and done to: Recognition theory, intersubjectivity and the third*. Routledge.

Black, M. J. (2003). Enactment: Analytic musings on energy, language, and personal growth. *Psychoanalytic Dialogues*, *13*(5), 633–655.

Bromberg, P. M. (2010). Minding the dissociative gap. *Contemporary Psychoanalysis*, *46*(1), 19–31.

Fanon, F. (2004). *The wretched of the earth*, trans. R. Philcox. Grove.

Kamola, I. A. (2011). Pursuing excellence in a "world-class African university": The Mamdani affair and the politics of global higher education. *Journal of Higher Education in Africa*, *9*(1/2), 147–168.

Kamola, I. A. (2015). Steve Biko and a critique of global governance as white liberalism. *African Identities*, *13*(1), 62–76.

Kessi, S. (2013). Re-politicizing race in community development: Using postcolonial psychology and Photovoice methods for social change. *Psychology in Society*, *45*, 19–35.

Kessi, S. and Cornell, J. (2015). Coming to UCT: Black students, transformation and discourses of race. *Journal of Student Affairs in Africa*, *3*(2), 1–16.

Maldonado-Torres, N. (2016). *Outline of ten theses on coloniality and decoloniality*. Fondation Frantz Fanon.

Mamdani, M. (1998). Teaching Africa at the post-apartheid University of Cape Town: A critical view of the "Introduction to Africa" core course in the social science and humanities faculty's foundation semester, 1998. *Social Dynamics*, *24*(2), 1–32.

Mamdani, M. (2018). *The African university*. Retrieved 18 July 2018, from www.lrb.co.uk/v40/n14/mahmood-mamdani/the-african-university.

Ntsebeza, L. (2014). The Mafeje and the UCT saga: Unfinished business? *Social Dynamics*, *40*(2), 274–288.

Nyamnjoh, F. (2016). *# RhodesMustFall: Nibbling at resilient colonialism in South Africa*. Langaa.

Ogden, T. H. (2014). *Rediscovering psychoanalysis: Thinking and dreaming, learning and forgetting*. Routledge.
Orange, D. M. (2011). *The suffering stranger: Hermeneutics for everyday clinical practice*. Routledge.
Robins, S. (2014). Poo wars as matter out of place: "Toilets for Africa" in Cape Town. *Anthropology Today, 30*(1), 1–3.
Slochower, J. A. (2013). *Holding and psychoanalysis: A relational perspective*. Routledge.
Stern, D. B. (2013). *Unformulated experience: From dissociation to imagination in psychoanalysis* (Vol. *8*). Routledge.
Swartz, R. (2016). "Good citizens and gentlemen": Gender, reputation and identity at the South African college, 1880–1910. *South African Historical Journal, 68*(4), 517–535.
Swartz, S. (2007). The power to name: South African intersubjective psychoanalytic psychotherapy and the negotiation of racialized histories. *European Journal of Psychotherapy and Counselling, 9*(2), 177–190.
Swartz, S. (2012). The broken mirror: Difference and shame in South African psychotherapy. *International Journal of Psychoanalytic Self Psychology, 7*(2), 196–212.
Winnicott, D. W. (1965). *The maturational processes and the facilitating environment: Studies in the theory of emotional development*. Karnac.
Winnicott, D. W. (1969). The use of an object. *The International Journal of Psycho-Analysis, 50*, 711–716.
Winnicott, D. W. (2002). *Through paediatrics to psychoanalysis: Collected papers*. Karnac.

Chapter 7

Ruth and the missing middle

Conflicts between groups of people generate narratives in which polarized positions quickly crystalize and create versions of events that place their stamp on both material and subjective realities. In these situations, the conflicts, and the narratives describing them, are always inseparable; as our theory suggests, subjectivity and relationality are socially constructed through systems of representation (Swartz, 2007). Conflicts etch deeply the divisions between opposing groups, and each might be represented by the other as "centre" (holding power, for example) or "marginal" (being under erasure, victimized, deprived of power). It is a volatile dynamic in which centre and periphery change not only over the course of time, but also with alterations in standpoint. The centre/margin trope describes an intersubjective field dominated and constrained by a relatively stable and self-sustaining set of dynamics organized around contested positions of power, legitimacy and authority. One of its most significant features is the way it assumes, subsumes, weaves itself a whole field, dividing players into those "in" and those "out," perpetrators and victims, the powerful and the despised ranged against the powerless and the dispossessed – a coercive and compelling dynamic almost impossible to resist (Benjamin, 2004, 2013). This is the ruthlessness of object relating, in which each side single-mindedly forges a path through to destruction of its demonized counterpart (Winnicott, 1969, p. 713). However, as the margins contest the legitimacy and stability of the centre, and new centres and peripheries proliferate, identities fracture, and subjectivities connect and reconnect in ways that at times offer ways of looking beyond centre and margin, into the webs between, of obscurity and richness of the often undescribed middle, neither centre nor margin, and yet potentially critical to the construction of the third.

The centre/margin relationship, as it is being played out in the decolonial project on South African university campuses, has been responsible for surfacing successfully the bitterly divisive and racist legacy of British colonialism and apartheid, and has raised awareness about the ways in which knowledge and institutional hierarchies continue to rehearse old lines of colonial privilege. Although material conditions of learning (most critically, fee structures) have driven protests, the movement also has subjectivity at its heart: many students and workers have described eloquently their experience of black pain, a sense of alienation on campus, of their own lives and knowledges being rendered invisible through both content of courses and styles of teaching. It is a fierce contest, with conflicting positions fluidly in focus, each casting the shadows into which the missing middle falls.

The chapter describes several highly charged encounters in which the missing middle gave voice to this complex version of the third, created space for encounters that destabilized well-rehearsed enemy/ally positions, and provided, albeit briefly, new paths through embattled and trauma-laden experience. It uses these encounters to foreground ways in which relational theory might be used to think through the challenges presented by situations of polarized conflict (Boonzaier, 2014; Samuels, 2015). These include the significance of moments of meeting between opposing interlocutors and the potential to create active witnessing through the fluidity of the missing middle (Altman, 2011; Benjamin, 2011, 2016; Orange, 2006; Stern, 1998; Ullman, 2011). The chapter concludes by suggesting that creating spaces for thinking in traumatic situations of conflict sometimes depends on embracing contradiction and complexity, ambiguously and untidily held in the middle ground.

The argument in this paper assumes as its foundation the work of Jessica Benjamin and Pumla Gobodo-Madikizela, particularly their work on witnessing in societies divided by long-standing conflict. It takes up in particular the role of witnessing in mitigating the traumatic effects of conflict (Benjamin, 2004; Gobodo-Madikizela, 2008). It also raises questions around the definition and boundaries of conflict. In a community divided, all are touched by conflict, but in different ways, and to different degrees. For some, engaging the conflict is central to daily life and a preoccupation; for others, it is but one strand of many conflicts, all preoccupying; yet others are dimly aware of trouble but pass by on the other side of the road. In refusing a solitary master narrative that insists on the singularity and overarching salience of a conflict dynamic, many conflicts and many narratives emerge in a complex relationship, and these in turn foster diversity in the act of witnessing itself. The question then becomes: to what am I witness?

There are three points critical to my argument in this chapter. First, I am arguing that those not directly constellated as players in the central conflict intersect with the intersubjective field in ways that constitute a vantage point from outside the dyad. This is one formulation of thirdness (Aron, 1999; Benjamin, 2017, p. 23). Second, those caught between complementary poles, not on one side or another, and attempting to maintain the ordinary routines that the conflict disrupts, hold a transitional space in which the terms of the central conflict might be ignored, played out, discarded or embraced, in a constantly changing dynamic. It offers, therefore, intersubjective fields that overlap with the central conflict but have degrees of freedom to experiment with multiple perspectives. This view of thirdness echoes Benjamin's formulation of the third not as a reified "thing," but a relationship (Benjamin, 2017, p. 23). It is important to note that the operation of either submission or surrender is complicated for the muddled middle, which is not asked explicitly to do either (see Benjamin, 2017, p. 24). In this sense, it is a transitional space with a fluid set of identities hallucinated by both sides. The question I am raising is about the kinds of affect being laundered in this space, the effects on those caught in their waves, and their significance for those locked into complementarity. Finally, I use this description of the missing middle as a way of elaborating on the environment surrounding conflict as essential to going-on-being, to the stage that allows conflict to be sought and embodied. Here, I draw on Winnicott's description of setting, in "Metapsychological and Clinical Aspects of Regression," as essential to analytic work (Winnicott, 2002, p. 278).

Protests in bounded communities

As described in previous chapters, from 2015, many South African universities have found themselves confronting a demand from students and workers that they transform. This is not a demand for slow change that honours tradition while responding sensitively to a changing social context. South African university traditions are in fact in the eye of the storm, saturated as they are with a legacy of colonial oppression and a model of knowledge hierarchies drawn largely from northern hemisphere scholarship. The student movement specifically is asking for decolonized free education; this very directly raises issues about curricula, and what is taught by whom, as well as issues around the financial models that have sustained the operation of universities to this point. The demand for decolonization goes hand in hand with workers' demands for better working conditions. Taken together, the student/worker movement has dared to imagine universities as communities within which the promises of post-apartheid South Africa might be realized. The past two years have confronted us all with fundamental questions: the autonomy of universities and academic freedom; the role of the state in subsidizing university education for students unable to afford it; the African continent as centre, not margin, in the world of research and knowledge production; and underlying it all, the very nature of a university as a site for thinking and dialogue.

While South African universities' turmoil expresses conflict, disappointment and hope peculiar to South Africa, with its colonial and apartheid history, and ongoing disparities in access to material and social security, it also has resonated with global struggles against class and race privilege, gender violence, and distortion in what constitutes "teachable" knowledge. Universities are a conduit between local and international scholarship, and insofar as they embrace diversity in their policies of admission they also bring together staff and students from different class, cultural and social positions. Residential universities are bounded communities: the extent of diversity in their populations is immediately visible in lecture theatres and avenues, in senate meetings and student rallies. Just as significantly, protest, when it happens, has an impact on everyone in the community, regardless of an individual's social or political identity, or place in the university machinery. Lines of loyalty to "the university" and commitment to it as a prized part of a social identity, founded perhaps on the ideals of debate, wisdom, knowledge generation and transmission, further bind members in. Universities are, after all, supposed to be spaces of thinking and reflection, fearless research and writing, selfless devotion to an investment in societies' newest generation of scholars; they are not greedy corporations or mindless government bureaucracies. All of this affects the ways in which universities ask for membership.

The ways in which protest movements might play out in bounded communities was brought to life in the 2015 and 2016 protests on the University of Cape Town's campus. The Rhodes Must Fall protests and their immediate aftermath brought together large and often festive crowds that appeared to foster in many excitement, hope and belief in the transformation project as both achievable and essential. As the management and protesters continued to clash, and the ongoing academic project was threatened, mass meetings gave way to protest of a different kind. Highly mobile groups of students occupied buildings, led marches, blockaded roads, took over executive and management meetings, set off fire alarms, interrupted lectures, and turned staff and students out of offices and classrooms. At times, teaching on campus came to a halt, and all but key operations were put on hold, as the university executive and student leaders met with mediators in a series of tense negotiations, frequently live-streamed to the university community. There were many rough and traumatic encounters, sometimes involving private security and police. Cars were set alight, doors broken into. While not peaceful, the protests were also often not overtly violent, although violence was a constant threat, and experienced by many as imminent.

Change as a result of this has been swift and wide-ranging. We live now in a landscape transformed: rules and hierarchies of power have undergone a radical shift, curricula are being rethought, and fee structures debated nationally, in and beyond universities. It is too early to say with any certainty where we will be in 5 or 10 years, but the rupture with the past has been made, and like all ruptures this profound there is much repair work to be done. This is not a fabric to be stitched together again; the fabric itself must be manufactured anew. My concern in this chapter is to reflect on the effects of these shifts on staff and students bound in to the university by job descriptions or registration for degrees, identified with it as in many respects a highly respected institution of higher learning, and with varying political views and personal aspirations, and yet finding themselves subject to a disorienting degree of change.[1]

Constituting the missing middle

In situations of polarizing conflict, the extreme positions are in plain view, and are plainly expressed in a kind of "if you're not for us, you're against us" division, which is rehearsed in action, attack and defence, and the representation of both in statements, minutes, posters and banners, headlines and tweets. The bifurcation often renders members of the community in conflict as necessarily belonging to one camp or the other. It is in order to complicate this binary that I am focusing on community members that for various reasons cannot be interpellated in this way. Many had not declared their views on the protests in any public way, except insofar as their work was directly affected. Within the bounds of job description, course requirements, laboratory, cleaning or office duties, they continued to show up for work; when interrupted, they departed for home, where some continued to work online. Even as the rules of work changed on their screens, in their encounters with line managers, tutors and lecturers, this large body of men and women maintained a steady eye on the goals as they saw them, and as defined by highly variable priorities and pressures, only some of which could be attributable to the earthquake shaking the university's foundations. They were from every part of the university community: kitchen and cleaning staff in residences, students at every level, administrators and receptionists, and academic and research staff. I am not suggesting that lack of affiliation to one or other side of the conflict was stable over time; it was not. As particular events unfolded, many had opinions for a time that identified them with one side or the other. But these affiliations were fluid and could change as contexts changed, and were in some way parallel to daily goals rather than determinative of them. The contrast here is with members of management or student leaders for whom the protests shaped daily goals.

Within the group I am casting as being in the middle, many found themselves in the front line of the conflict, in that they were placed in a no man's land between management and student leaders or protesting workers. Some held positions that were in the ranks of line management, and, depending on where they sat in the university hierarchy, were expected to implement university policy, despite personal opinions about it. This situation was ambiguous, or – to put it more bluntly – confused and confusing. Some of the staff worked vigorously in meetings to argue for fundamental policy change, and when this was not forthcoming, implemented policy they saw as problematic. Some waited for clarity on what the rules might become. Some devoted themselves to a task that swiftly emerged as urgent: that of containing the anxiety in their staff and students about the tumult the whole community was experiencing.

I had access to line managers and many other staff during times of protest through my position as a faculty management executive. My portfolio was to look after staffing matters. During the protests, I found myself encountering a wide range of feelings in staff at every level, from outrage, hardening racist attitudes and fear, through to active sympathy for and collaboration with the change project. Depending on what those staff brought to encounters with me in terms of previous experiences, knowledge of my political views and ways of working, hopes for and suspicion of management, I became enemy or ally, or something in between, a receptacle for anxiety, and wearer of projections, a failing protector, capacious container, demon whisperer and maker of impromptu rules. My own experiences of my shifting subjectivity I have described in detail in earlier work, and I will not rehearse it here (Swartz, 2012, 2016). Rather, the argument I want to develop arises from attempts of many in positions similar to mine to craft a role in relation to a community of people in need of all kinds of practical and emotional support. There was a need for accountability to their immediate physical and emotional welfare, a kind of ambulance service, offering bandages and temporary transport to quieter spaces. Being a witness to emergency states would mean at times bracketing some personal beliefs (Slochower, 2013). To be helpful at all demanded openness and emotional availability. The balance of bracketing and authentic presence in volatile conditions is always necessarily precarious. Moreover, to assume that ambulance runs are welcome and helpful rather than intrusive, presumptuous and clumsy had constantly to be borne in mind.

All around was conflict and chaos. We often did not know what the day would bring. Colleagues in departmental units, comrades assigned to particular projects, and friends tracked events obsessively through WhatsApp groups, tweets and Facebook. There were crisis meetings through evenings and weekends. Many of us moved through buildings, in and out of offices, along the avenues, watching and listening, aware of escalating trauma on all sides as confrontations intensified. We faced the imminent collapse of the academic schedule, and along with it the possibility of graduating final-year students and making possible the intake of a new cohort of students.

But what exactly were we being a witness to? Of course, there were the poles of the conflict and the contours of their battle starkly represented in contradictory narratives endlessly cancelling each other, a swirl of rumour and versions of events attested to as facts. There were also many fissures opened by that conflict – gender-based violence, racism, blinkered protection of class interests. It would be easy to represent everything we saw and heard as subsumed by the overarching context: to assert that in battle zones, every truth, every identity, every intersubjective field is subject to and dominated by the war – held hostage to a single narrative. But that would simplify and erase – fictionalize, even – a texture that hobbled between routine activities and a violent departure from them. Between zones, in and out of front lines, beyond the dissociated space of no man's land, there were many stories, many truths, and worlds of complexity, contradiction and ambiguity. We were witnessing many-sidedness.

In the vignettes that follow, I describe a series of encounters with staff navigating their way through this multiplicity. These staff members were caught somewhere between the poles of conflict, in the confusing, tearing middle, and I was being asked to bear witness to this confusion of identities.

Encounters

During the period I am describing, some academic staff were working from home, and as a result many of my encounters were with administrators, some angry with management, some with the protesters, some reporting panic attacks and nightmares, some looking detached and eerily calm. The conversations ranged widely, from matters of personal safety and daily challenges, through to comments on national and global politics. In some buildings, it was clear that administrators had taken over the role of looking after the welfare of both staff and students: they commanded their terrain fiercely and with authority. In others, administrators hid behind locked doors and cried out in alarm when there was a knock on the door. Occasionally, I came across a cluster, mainly of women – academic and administrative staff – sharing tea or lunch, elaborating on the latest news and rumours. They tested their predictions on me, and then sometimes fell into picking up comfortable conversations about an outside life unruptured by this immediate breakdown: weather, children, dogs and cats, the timing of their next holiday. All were deeply affected by the protests, but just as much with what had been before, and what must come after, in terms of completing the academic year – the detail of assignments, marks, examinations, students' ongoing ups and downs. These staff members' struggles with fear, anxiety and anger were articulated in part through the narrative of the protests, with each individual positioned uniquely in relation to it. At the same time, the lurch from day to day underscored an experience of erasure, insignificance and unprotected vulnerability. It was a wrenching perspective on an intersection of gender, race, class and power that had been largely hidden in the protest discourse.

As I walked through a building lobby, heading towards a group of approaching protesters, some students and some workers, on the main university avenue, I found two of the building's cleaners, a man and a woman. Both were agitated; they lingered under the stairwell in the shadows. I knew them both and stopped to ask how they were. There followed a babble of distressed talk. Some student protesters were demanding that the cleaners down tools as the protest movement had always embraced their working conditions and pay as part of what needed to change. They told me that their supervisors, following instruction from their own managers, were insisting they stay at work or they would be fired. Yes, they said, they supported the protest movement the year before, and their contracts had been changed as a result, from being with an agency external to the university to being with the university itself. But now the students were threatening to beat them because the whole university must be shut down. Then followed a tale they had heard of a student rumoured to have chased one of their team working in another building with a mop. Knowing that I was part of the academic executive in that part of the university, they wanted my advice on what to do. Responding to anxiety strongly expressed in that moment, I arranged that the supervisors be called, and that they located a room in which to make themselves a cup of tea. In a subsequent meeting of staff from various sectors, all involved in some way with the cleaning staff's circumstances and contracts, a plan was made for the coming days, which it was hoped would protect those who felt caught in a conflict they did not wish to take part in themselves.

This was a moment of deep complexity, one in which class and lack of access to material resources and privilege set this man and woman up against a protest movement purporting to be fighting, partly at least, in their name. For the two cleaning staff I encountered, there had been an appropriation of identity to be one with the "student/worker" struggle, and yet both had a loyalty to the staff in the building they took care of. Their long connection to various inhabitants of the building's offices was displayed over and over in shared jokes and news of children and holidays, worry about ailing relatives, and irritation with disrespectful waste and mess.

To be cleaning up after the privileged, to be emptying dustbins rather than filling them up, is a relationship iconic of the exploitation of black labour by colonial oppressors, and points very directly to class differences in a society that does not assume that those with resources should clean up after themselves. Despite the irreducibility of this, the encounter opened a perspective on multiple locations of subjectivity, and the ways in which this might offer the emergence of moments of meeting.

Later the same day, the executive dean of the faculty and I followed in the wake of a small band of protesters as they went from building to building. They sang, shouted and drummed. One had a stick that he used to beat on locked office doors.

Despite cancellation of lectures, departmental administrators were expected to come in, and to continue the work of answering emails, managing departmental grants and funds, keeping the shreds of the usual cycle of course assignments and examinations in whatever order they could impose. Unlike their academic colleagues, this group of staff had no freedom to choose whether to work at home or come to campus: a personnel department that in ordinary times watched unauthorized absence from work vigilantly seemed ambivalent about where to put their weight, behind staff safety or adherence to rules. In the absence of clarity, they assumed presence. Many departmental administrators came to work each morning, long journeys for some, only to find their building inaccessible, doors locked, and little guidance from their academic line managers. Moreover, unlike the cleaners, the university's administrators never had an explicitly laid out stake in the protest. Largely silent on the public stage, and squeezed between academic staff, on the one side, and the students whose work towards their degrees they administered, on the other, they found themselves on 100 front lines, day by day, fielding anxious calls from students inside and outside of the protest movement, angry and frustrated parents, academics asking for online work to be completed, and protesters demanding they down tools.

One man, in charge of administering a busy undergraduate programme for his department, took me aside, and, wringing his hands, asked whether he could please come in to work at night, rather than face another day of bruising encounters in his building. As the only male member of his team, he said he had felt he should protect his female co-workers and shield them when he was able to. But now, he said, his health was failing. He was having nightmares every night. Here was a man burdened both by having constructed the protesters as violent and dangerous, and by being constructed as "the man of the house," called to stand up to the hyper-masculinity on display in the those tasked with making sure work in every university building was interrupted for the day. In the double assault, he made an extraordinary offer to switch his night and day, offering me a glimpse not only into the multiplicities of identity, but also of trauma being surfaced even in the conflict's outer eddies.

In the same building, but another department, a woman working behind a locked door burst into tears when I asked her how she was. Without information, I assumed, as she wiped her tears, that her stress was the result of trying to work day after day in stressful conditions, and in her case with academic line managers who chose often not to come to campus. While these assumptions were correct as far as they went, they described only a small part of her anger and anxiety. Strongly identified with the student movement politically, she was enraged by what she saw as management's recalcitrance. At the same time, students confided in her, and many wanted to complete the academic year, despite the protest movement's insistence that a sacrifice needed to be made. She was also protective of her head of department and wanted to manage administrative deadlines for his sake. With lines of loyalty pulling at her, she furiously rejected my question, and it appeared in the moment that she, not surprisingly, identified me with a kind of false care sometimes promoted in organizations as good for productivity. Without seeing with her own eyes that I was with her, she assumed I was against her, and she told me angrily that she preferred not to talk about her feelings.

A third administrator recounted an event in which protesters tried to break into a locked section of a department, believing there to be staff at work despite the call for university closure. A colleague had arrived on the scene and managed to defuse the situation by reassuring students that everyone in that corridor would leave the building immediately. In telling me the story, the administrator said over and over that she was unable to recall the number of emergency services in the heat of the moment. This captured her flood of anxiety, and her sense of shame that she had been protected and had failed herself to protect. She was not herself an emergency service, she could not be reached. Unlike the woman I had seen immediately before, she had no strong views about the protests themselves, but with a sudden sense that she had failed in how she defined her "duty," she slipped into traumatic repetition.

I turn now to another version of the middle ground. With colleagues, I sat next to a lecturer relatively new to the faculty. He had supported the university closure and been a close ally of the protesters. He had encouraged students and tutors in their wish to boycott the few lectures still running. Having encountered police brutality in previous years, he was clear that he would find it abhorrent to come to campus if lectures were resumed with a strong security presence to prevent disruption. We had little more than a brief acquaintance, and he had no reason to trust that I would be helpful. In the meeting, he was largely silent. When I talked, he turned his head to eye me flatly, unblinkingly, and with disconcerting unwillingness to make himself a part of the rhythm of the exchanges happening around him. I left the meeting with a strong feeling of discovering myself wearing the clothes of an enemy that he had tossed my way. There was a way in which this was a truth I needed to own. I was wearing enemy clothes, in the sense that during the meeting I had more than once referred to my responsibilities as part of the executive team. "Wearing a hat" of a particular sort in this context was to identify with the management enemy, but the image of being able to don different hats also signalled a form of privilege, a freedom to choose between roles, that many of my interlocutors did not have. I was referring to a worry about tutors' contracts, and the possibilities of moulding these to fit extraordinary circumstances, and also to the effect on a limited budget of extending contracts beyond the academic calendar year. These concerns made explicit my role as part management, and in this instance the way in which the encounter positioned him and I as enemies jolted me into seeing myself through his eyes. I walked away uncomfortably double, in ways that I describe in more detail in Chapter 5.

A week later, with students and staff both in and beyond the protest movement facing the implications of a collapsing academic year, escalating student loans, and agitating families, the lecturer and I found ourselves in another meeting. He was torn between his loyalty to the decolonial project, which asked for all to down pens, and the urgent pleas from students for lecture material, cobbled-together make-up tutorials, and the opportunity to write exams. Still not an ally, I now encountered his anxiety and the depth of the dilemma more rawly. Instead of the flat gaze, his eyes jumped back and forth, skittering across my face and back to his lists, his plans. I suppose neither of us felt safe. We seemed both to be finding our way, unscaffolded by any side we could join, no shelter in self-evident rights and justice. In this moment, there were only echoes of student voices: "I must earn money next year, so I must write my exams"; "my sister had a baby last month and needs me at home"; "my parents are gone, my grandmother is old, and has sacrificed for me to finish." It is these individual testimonies, and the call to hold an ethical position in relation to them, that carried the capacity to infest the conversation with anxiety to an extent that the polarizing discourses from opposing sides did not. He and his students were fractured not over the activist programme, but the meaning of sacrifice for individual students, and his role in bearing witness to every story. The path forward was littered with accusations of betrayal and desperate appeals for rescue. What he wanted from me in this was limited, and he continued to underscore his wariness because of my management position. He wished to craft his own way forward, story by story, and to help colleagues piece together something that would honour the protests, but also the needs of supplicants. With colleagues, I was being called on to provide a bureaucratic setting in which the fewest possible rules got in the way of his solutions. Work in this meeting became a version of thirdness – rule-moulding, oiling bureaucratic wheels – that both crafted me as "management enemy" but also drew me into a set of subversions of the letter of the law. While my experience was that we did not share any moments of affective resonance, our dilemmas mirrored each other, and that was a symmetry with which I was able to move internally away from identifying myself simply as matter out of place (Douglas, 2003).

There is one final vignette with which to illustrate the complex subjectivities surrounding the protests. From time to time, I was a part of meetings at the university's wellness and counselling centre. This is a service that provides short-term psychotherapy and counselling to registered students. It was conceived originally as the kind of counselling provision that would meet the needs of a young adult and academically talented population. Resources in terms of budget and staffing were designed to meet the needs of a student body imagined as in general likely to cope emotionally, with the slightest of nudges needed occasionally to get back on track. More serious mental illness would be referred out of the university, to state or private service providers, depending on the families' means. The resources on offer were never going to be adequate (and there is, of course, an argument to be made that it is not the university's place to provide an encompassing mental health service for its student body). In South Africa, the usual challenges being faced around the tumult of entering into a new phase of life are compounded for many by complicated histories of familial, political and social trauma, caused by decades of oppression, displacement, poverty and endemic violence, including high rates of sexual assault. Even before the protests, the resources of the mental health professionals at the centre were challenged by the extent and depth of trauma in the students they saw; once the protests began, the triggering effect of rallies and clashes between students and security police and members of staff raised an affective hurricane. They began to receive unprecedented levels of complaint from all sides. Academic staff were frustrated that the counselling service was unable to respond quickly enough to situations of crisis and trauma that unfolded daily on campus and in residences; complaints about unavailability and inefficiency were endlessly rehearsed in meetings. Some student activists accused counsellors of inaccessibility, and of being too enmeshed with northern hemisphere ways of approaching psychiatry and psychotherapy to understand the roots and nature of black pain. Several student suicides and suicide attempts fuelled a public discourse of complaint.

The counsellors saw students from all sides of the struggle. Some students suffered with extreme anxiety and other symptoms of post-traumatic stress after brutal encounters with police and security. Some students said that they were pressurized into joining the protest movement by those with whom they shared residence space. Some were also being rebuked for not studying by worried parents. A few came for counselling after they had been caught up with moments of crowd violence. And in and around the uproar of the protests, a steady stream of students were subjected to sexual harassment or violence. The new demand was over and above an already full load.

At the time of the protests, and in recognition of the levels of trauma being caused, or being caused to surface from the past, by ongoing waves of highly charged encounters, management alerted all students to the service's availability to those feeling distressed, even if the university closed its academic programme. At the same time, the psychologists were told they come to work "at their own risk." Their building was vulnerable – just down the road, buildings had been occupied and cars set alight. They occasionally struggled to concentrate, jumped at loud noises during our meetings, and glanced anxiously towards the windows whenever there was a movement outside. Their sympathies as citizens of the university community had often been with the protesters, but here in their daily work they saw and heard all the costs on every side. They created moments of holding. Their loyalties were torn. They held unbearable secrets, crimes and punishments, escalating racial divides, hatred collapsing into terror, and took it in, contained and reflected it, and became more grey.

As professionals, the student counsellors were being asked to imagine themselves into many subjectivities, to reflect fractured versions of events, to stretch empathy in ways we seldom imagine we could. And yet in the shape-shifting and in the constant questioning of identities, inside and out, there emerged a cohesive core, a witnessing, not just of the conflict, or the trauma it produces, but the bewildering complexity of a total situation (Joseph, 1985). The poles were there to be seen, but were solidly rooted in a world of experiences between. My own role was often to be a sounding board not about individual cases as much as the functioning of the team as a whole, its resourcefulness in fighting off the position of abjection so constantly on offer through the voices of critics, and to celebrate cohesion in the face of fracture elsewhere.

Reflections on the middle as third

Conflict on South African university campuses revisits the terrible and lasting effects of both apartheid and colonialism, a legacy of racial injustice and dehumanization. Decolonizing universities has taken the student movement into a direct struggle with unearned privilege, the legitimacy and authority of scholarship cast as "fact" or "truth," lines of power embedded in rules and traditions, workers' rights, and a myriad of social justice issues around race, class and gender discrimination and violence. Transformation has been abrupt, disruptive and patchy, and we are between places, in some respects a divided community, resonating on every level with some unmetabolized trauma. We are still being shaped by a discourse in public settings that too often falls back on the celebration of heroes and denigration of villains, guilt, victimhood and denial. There have been many witnesses actively involved battle by battle, and of course many bystanders.

However long the road ahead, and whatever its contours, the work of building resilience into an always-collapsing third must exercise us, not only for the sake of healing a riven community, but also to enable universities to serve their purpose, to sponsor creativity, open debate, curiosity and play. There is also the possibility to be explored that this context might have the potential to shed light on other conflicts, on protest movements, situations of oppression and opposition, and demands for transformation.

In the past few years, I have seen the complexity for those on both sides of the conflict of being fully engaged witnesses. It demands extraordinary emotional presence, vulnerability and tolerance of challenge to achieve a secure sense of an identity that gives legitimacy to the witnessing role. Moreover, the role of reconstituting the third as it collapses internally, with the self split by persecutory anxiety and tugged into fight or flight, is constant, and does not stop once the talking ends.

What I have been exploring here is at a slant to this: it is neither separate from nor assimilable into activities involving direct engagement with negotiating the protests and the changes they bring about, or witnessing of this process. I am describing a witnessing, but it is of the swirl of people and routines, displacements and worries of a whole community in upheaval. The vignettes I have offered in this chapter are about unsettlement and identity dispersal, players driven by widely differing views, loyalties, economic imperatives and skills. Each showed me another surface of a multi-surfaced and constantly moving globe. In this middle, we have to tolerate confusion and collision of contradictory narratives to hold two minds in order to muddle towards some kind of recognizing exchange. Life in this ambiguous ground builds and rebuilds a perspective that resists collapse into complementarity, simply through an immersion in the waywardness of truths.

There are three ways in which the idea of ruthlessness and its relationship to the third is illuminated by an immersion in muddled middle ground. The first concerns the ruthlessness of large institutions, which are structured by rules applied in necessarily relentless ways. Winnicott might have referred to this kind of ruthlessness as one aspect of "hate" in psychoanalysis, for example in the imposition of time limits to sessions and payment of fees, those fixed rules that establish the container within which the flux of relationship plays itself out (see Winnicott, 2002, p. 285).

Protest movements on South African campuses significantly disrupted the container over and over, but there were many ways in which routines of academic activity kept reasserting themselves for everyone, on both sides of the conflict. Protesting students and staff as groups demanded universities' temporary closure as part of a confrontation with management, and while there were sometimes threats that buildings might be burned down, the setting itself held, including the materiality of ways buildings hold space in particular ways. This includes the organization of people's work within those spaces. Rules and procedures, even though contested, insisted on continuity. They became a place to start from. If the rules and procedures protected forms of colonial privilege, what form might new rules take? The protests returned again and again to the demand that the rules be changed, sometimes in radical ways. Significantly, as a community, we became self-conscious about rules and the need for rules, in ways that were previously part of an unthought known (Bollas, 2017).

I am suggesting here that the idea of a university, and a general commitment to its purpose (to offer higher education in the form of degrees), was an indispensable structure that enabled an unfolding of a group dynamic explosive in its intent. The university, even when apparently deserted by day, or fractured by turbulence, remained "reliably there, on time, alive, breathing" (Winnicott, 2002, p. 285). This quality of survival was invested across an army of people, each of whom played a role in keeping simple routines remembered, a setting recognizable and a future imaginable. In a similar way, a patient might rage at a therapist and demand fundamental change to the therapeutic relationship, but still be soothed by the regularity of arranged sessions, the unchanging constellation of furniture in the room, the familiarity of the way in and out of the building. The ruthlessness of the setting – broadly defined – and the steadiness of all those that attended minutely to it underwrote the possibility of change being made meaningful. To reiterate the paradox Winnicott draws attention to, it was the ruthless attack on the object, the hated colonial edifice, the pile of rules of privilege, that eventually underwrote its survival and ensured survivability as a future. A chaotic level of change was held – and celebrated – within the embrace of the idea of a university as a rule-bound community.

Second, the mid-field muddle, the unsettled many in the midst of turmoil, created a third as a place of observation. Deeply affected by disruption, and yet not called on to strategize, make public statements, march or argue with either side, freed many in the university community to notice the contours of the conflict, to predict its shape day by day, and reach for a place of reflection and planning even when feelings ran high. By its nature, the muddled middle embraced many points of view; it also by definition therefore was not aligned to one side or the other of the conflict. Irreducible multiplicity makes for a sturdy third.

It would be erroneous to cast the middle as a group of relatively anonymous, faceless and voiceless bystanders, or even witnesses, although individuals played the roles of both from time to time. My experience, talking to those I have characterized as working in and around the central lines of polarization, was that there was talk and action, dissociation and passivity, witnessing and acts of compassion and heroism, none of which could be easily subsumed in the conflict's dominant narratives. Where there was sufficient safety, the middle space appeared to operate successfully as a transitional space, one in which fantasies of revenge and rescue might be voiced, trauma rehearsed, anger and anxiety vented. It was a space in which old routines were nostalgically revisited, and new ones excitedly practised and shared. Perhaps most significantly, this part of the third was alive with experimentation, a trying on of new roles and points of view. As agents in busy communities, they were involved in countless acts of submission and surrender, as we all are all the time. The conditions of both of these warrant further discussion.

For example, the missing middle staff were frequently asked to submit to the university's demand that they attend work regardless of protest activity on campus. This ruling was flouted by many in line management positions, who allowed staff to leave work early, or work from home, when this seemed appropriate. To be "given permission" to be absent from campus, against the ruling of central management, by someone lower on the hierarchy seemed to build in another layer of submission, this time to a mindful manager. In reality, this was a process of deferral, delegation and negotiation, in which "permissions" were sought, taken up, ignored and reworded daily. What I encountered very frequently was not submission, but subversion, and this seems to me to add to the possibilities of building a third space.

In terms of surrender, I saw in many individuals a grappling with lines of personal accountability to individual staff and students, and indeed to the total situation (Joseph, 1985). It was as if protest had thrown everything up in the air, old identities, ways of seeing the world. Those with the resources to do so used fluidity to craft new approaches to old problems, some of which were related directly to protest action, and many of which were brushing the dust out of ordinary dysfunctional routines. Over and over, I heard staff commenting on the rupture with the past. They were experiencing their surrender to finding new ways to inhabit jobs both confusing and enlivening. In some respects, what was being done each day mimicked the old, and followed habitual routines, but there was a demand that every task, every day, be carried out with a different consciousness of its significance. This was critical in the sense that a colonial situation reproduces itself mechanically, with application of rules and regulations mindlessly impacting those with the least access to privilege.

Note

1 I have disguised the identity of individuals throughout this chapter to protect their anonymity.

References

Altman, N. (2011). Response to Chana Ullman's paper "Between denial and witnessing." *Psychoanalytic Perspectives*, *8*(2), 201–206.

Aron, L. (1999). Clinical choices and the relational matrix. *Psychoanalytic Dialogues*, *9*(1), 1–29.

Benjamin, J. (2004). Beyond doer and done to: An intersubjective view of thirdness. *The Psychoanalytic Quarterly*, *73*(1), 5–46.

Benjamin, J. (2011). Acknowledgment of collective trauma in light of dissociation and dehumanization. *Psychoanalytic Perspectives*, *8*(2), 207–214.

Benjamin, J. (2013). *The bonds of love: Psychoanalysis, feminism, & the problem of domination*. Pantheon.

Benjamin, J. (2016). Non-violence as respect for all suffering: Thoughts inspired by Eyad El Sarraj. *Psychoanalysis, Culture & Society*, *21*(1), 5–20.

Benjamin, J. (2017). *Beyond doer and done to: Recognition theory, intersubjectivity and the third*. Routledge.

Boonzaier, F. (2014). South African women resisting dominant discourse in narratives of violence. In M. N. Lafrance and S. McKenzie-Mohr (Eds.), *Women voicing resistance: Discursive and narrative explorations* (pp. 102–120). Routledge.

Bollas, C. (2017). *The shadow of the object: Psychoanalysis of the unthought known*. Routledge.

Douglas, M. (2003). *Purity and danger: An analysis of concepts of pollution and taboo*. Routledge.

Gobodo-Madikizela, P. (2008). Trauma, forgiveness and the witnessing dance: Making public spaces intimate. *Journal of Analytical Psychology*, *53*(2), 169–188.

Joseph, B. (1985). Transference: The total situation. *International Journal of Psychoanalysis*, *66*(4), 447–454.

Orange, D. M. (2006). For whom the bell tolls: Context, complexity, and compassion in psychoanalysis. *International Journal of Psychoanalytic Self Psychology*, *1*(1), 5–21.

Samuels, A. (2015). *The political psyche*. Routledge.

Slochower, J. A. (2013). *Holding and psychoanalysis: A relational perspective*. Routledge.

Stern, D. (1998). Non-interpretive mechanisms in psychoanalytic therapy: The "something more" than interpretation. *The International Journal of Psycho-Analysis*, *79*(5), 903–921.

Swartz, S. (2007). The power to name: South African intersubjective psychoanalytic psychotherapy and the negotiation of racialized histories. *European Journal of Psychotherapy and Counselling*, *9*(2), 177–190.

Swartz, S. (2012). The broken mirror: Difference and shame in South African psychotherapy. *International Journal of Psychoanalytic Self Psychology*, *7*(2), 196–212.

Swartz, S. (2016). *Rhodes, falling*. Paper presented at the IARRP annual conference, Rome, 2016.

Ullman, C. (2011). Between denial and witnessing: Psychoanalysis and clinical practice in the Israeli context. *Psychoanalytic Perspectives*, *8*(2), 179–200.
Winnicott, D. W. (1969). The use of an object. *The International Journal of Psycho-Analysis*, *50*, 711–716.
Winnicott, D. W. (2002). *Through paediatrics to psychoanalysis: Collected papers*. Karnac.

Chapter 8

Decolonizing psychoanalysis

Liable to inherit

Psychoanalysis has a long history in South Africa (Hayes, 2008; Raphael-Leff, 2016). Its presence is remarkable because of the absence particularly during the apartheid years of regular contact with international colleagues, and the steady emigration of those wanting to pursue their training in psychoanalytic centres in the United Kingdom and the United States. We became for a time a community largely self-taught and tenuously maintained with papers and texts that came to us through libraries, visits abroad and occasional workshops with international elders in the long years before the transition to democracy. There was no opportunity in this situation to throw ourselves ruthlessly at psychoanalytic parents and to emerge with survival secure. We were dealing with absence, in which fantasies of the power and wisdom of idealized authority fed a sense of abandonment, inadequacy and persecutory anxiety about our (il)legitimacy. Yet despite the lack of formal structures through which the teaching and training of psychoanalysis might have been carried as both philosophy and practice, it never lost its influence.

Psychoanalytic practice has been consistently challenged in South Africa as having failed to prove its credentials as "evidence-based" and "solution-focused" (Kagee, 2006). Psychoanalytic psychotherapy is largely unavailable to the majority of South Africans in need of mental health interventions. Its slow unfolding over years rather than months is expensive and unsustainable for individuals and families for whom short-term relief is urgent. Further, its reputation as being irrelevant because of its lack of rootedness in an African context has been cemented by its identification over decades with white middle-class practitioners and clients (Ruane, 2010). Its persistent presence has thus become a marker of the obduracy of white privilege.

An explanation for the continuing influence of psychoanalysis through South Africa's desert years probably lies in what we have been, in Mannoni's resonant phrase, "liable to inherit" (Mannoni, 1972, quoted in Brickman, 2003, p. 490). We – psychoanalytic psychotherapists and teachers – inherited through a number of charismatic teachers, and also through exchanges between psychoanalytic kin reaching across the seas. Certainly, teacherly DNA, handed from one generation of clinical trainers to the next, had the effect of sustaining the legacy of Freud in this diaspora, most significantly through the psychoanalytic slant of clinical psychology programmes in major universities (Swartz, 2007b). In this, the shaping effect of psychoanalytically trained ex-South Africans who maintained ties with colleagues cannot be underestimated. It remains a powerful form of transmission, keeping the psychoanalytic baby alive.

The traces from teacher to pupil are relatively easy to map, but the nature of these interrupted "tense and tender ties" (Stoler, 2001) is an insufficient explanation for the lusty desire to maintain the psychoanalytic project against the odds. The argument that follows unpacks the complexity of what it means to inherit a body of theory with no indigenous roots, and the implications of this for the decolonial project.

The way that I am using the term "liable to inherit" in this argument is specific to the flow of knowledge from centres to colonized peripheries. In the context of a discussion of coloniality and psychoanalysis, it suggests at its most simple the transmission of knowledge from parent body to child body. It is a transmission, too, of attitudes towards the legitimate curriculum of psychoanalytic study, as well as a teaching and learning culture, dictating what should be taught, by whom, and in what kinds of settings. As with any inheritance, the child receives gifts, possibilities and problems. For those chafing against colonial authority, there is impingement, constant reminders that the colonial situation renders local originality as at most a curious addition to the centre's store of knowledge, but not a challenge to its foundational tenets. For those wanting to relegate the colonial situation to the past, there are problems with being recognized as legitimate adult kin. The dilemma might be posed as choosing between orphan status, and being in a boarding school, with limited access to the parental home. To extend the analogy, to decolonize psychoanalysis perhaps involves a choice between ambivalent dependency or casting oneself entirely as original, and therefore independent.

Psychoanalysis in South Africa began its life in a colonial situation, and its early years were inevitably shaped by the same complicity in othering black South Africans that characterized scientific racism (Dubow, 1995; Long, 2016b). Here is the unbroken strand of thought. During the years of Cape colonial rule, lunatic asylum superintendents were keen to describe "native mentality," assuming of course its difference from that of the settler population. This was the forerunner of an entire field of enquiry that was deeply influential throughout the British African colonies, for as long as they lasted (McCulloch, 1995; Swartz, 2015, 2017). So, for example, in 1895, lunatic asylum superintendent Dr T. D. Greenlees published a scientific paper describing the childish nature of black mentality; in it, he stated: "The native brain has its analogue in the European child's cerebrum; in many respects his mental attributes are similar to those of a child" (Greenlees, 1895, p. 75). He went to some lengths to provide evidence for this view through the study of the weight and appearance of the brains of black patients who had died in the asylum.

Decades later, Wulf Sachs' confirmation in *Black Hamlet* that his Rhodesian analysand John Chavafambira had a psyche susceptible to Freudian psychoanalytic understanding is equally imbued with a distinctly colonial curiosity, and has an assumption of difference (to be confirmed or denied) at its centre (Dubow, 1993; Long, 2017a; Sachs, 1937). These two instances map a repetition of a single colonial attitude, even as the shape of the discourse changed.

It is a discourse that refuses to go away. In 2017, during a tense discussion in one psychoanalytic reading group about the whiteness of much of the active South African psychoanalytic community, one participant suggested that psychoanalytic theory and practice are simply "irrelevant" to South Africa's black majority and black practitioners, in the sense perhaps of being of no interest, of not making sense. This was suggested as a reason for why we should not be surprised at the extent to which we continue to attract more white than black members. It was a statement disconcertingly close to the way successive colonial governments cast all but industrial schools as "irrelevant" to indigenous populations, arguing, for example, that to expose black students to literature was neither wanted or needed (Swartz, 2018).

It is a painful conundrum in two ways. First, the impulse among psychoanalytic psychotherapists to be immersed in cutting-edge theory coming from the centre underscores a colonial dependency and increases the danger of becoming "irrelevant" in grappling with our own political, social and economic context. Second, it speaks to a wish to be distanced from that part of the colonial situation, with its legacy of inequality, that carries a long history of saturation in discourses of difference (Long, 2016b, 2017a). Knowledge coming to this periphery from the centre is a kind of dissociative insulation from an emotionally challenging context.

I will be suggesting through the following sections that what we have been "liable to inherit" is shot through with this kind of ambivalence and complexity. There are two parts to the argument that follows. One concerns the intractability of the colonial past, and the traumatic ways in which it is repeated, and how these might contribute to efforts to find new ways to go forward. I will illustrate this by giving an extended example of what I have called "a colonial situation" to demonstrate repetitions of division and alienation with which we continue to wrestle. This is about a complicated doubleness of colonial relatedness, not only in relation to an international community that we imagine as casting us as colonial subjects without autonomy or confident access to an authentic and original voice, but also as local representatives of "colonial" settler government, embedded in a set of inherited object relations. The second part of the argument turns to the genealogy of primitivity and gender and race binaries as concepts running through foundational texts in psychoanalytic theory. Thinking through the implications of these concepts is essential for a decolonial project. The chapter will conclude with some thoughts about the contribution of the Winnicottian lens to undoing the colonial knottedness of psychoanalytic theory.

A colonial situation

It was the first international psychoanalytic conference to be held in South Africa after the transition to democracy. Entitled "Change: Psychoanalytic Perspectives," it was organized by the London-based South African Psychoanalysis Trust (SAPT) in 1998, largely compromising South African ex-patriots, in collaboration with South African-based mental health practitioners. According to Joan Raphael-Leff's brief account, the trust came together "with the singular aim of bringing South African psychoanalysis into line with international standards through the establishment of an accredited training institute" (Raphael-Leff, 2016). Conferences well attended by international psychoanalysts were presumably to be a part of this "bringing into line."

It was a generous reconnection after a period of alienation and exile, a sharing not only from the centre to the periphery of analytic wisdoms, but also a witnessing of the richness and diversity of the work of local practitioners. It was not set up to "school"; in fact, the respect with which the papers of local delegates were received was a tribute and a heartfelt witnessing of therapeutic work undertaken in often very difficult circumstances. Nonetheless, the flow from London of analysts to speak to a South African audience without official psychoanalytic credentials was inescapably and traumatically a repetition of the colonial situation. The danger of this repetition was acknowledged and reflected on at the time. One local delegate, Leslie Swartz, commented on the danger of bringing "the psychoanalytic exile home, internally," referring explicitly to a relationship of subjugation to the centre, the spectre haunting the event. He also asked ascerbically, "Why speak of the return of psychoanalysis? Psychoanalysis has never left" (reported in Ivey, 1998). An enactment, driven by these fierce affective currents, and carrying all the weight of unconscious impulse, shaped the course of events. This account will focus on two moments through which I hope to demonstrate the complexity of what was played out in 1998, and its connection to the meaning of decolonizing psychoanalysis now.

The conference programme was designed to be widely inclusive, celebrating diversity in practice, community and theory. The work of local practitioners, some working psychoanalytically and some not, all engaging with trauma, the devastating legacies of apartheid and under-resourcing on a massive scale, was approached with great care by the conference organizers, panel members and discussants. The work was honoured both within the space of conference discussion and also in ongoing contact once the conference was over.

There was perhaps no way to avoid the exoticization of "community work" in this context, or the constant signalling of a volatile set of binaries (those with resources and those without; those with the freedom to move between countries and those rooted to a single geography; those with psychoanalytic knowledge and those with little or none). These served as a rumbling backdrop to all that took place.

There were moments when the reactions of visiting psychoanalysts to the trauma they were being asked to stand witness to felt extremely helpful, particularly when it was related immediately and authentically to their own experience in a variety of UK contexts. This balancing across a potential us/them divide restored equilibrium, however briefly. More difficult were moments when visitors' reactions to traumatic displays of social and emotional trauma in community settings felt coloured with guilt around years of self-exile, or eagerness to "fill up" on intimate engagement that had been missed over the years.

There is no doubt that all we heard from the front lines of communities newly emerging from apartheid devastation was not simple to digest. It had no easy fit with traditional models of psychoanalytic practice. With those presenting having a very wide range of exposure to psychoanalytic theory, from plenty to none at all, even careful interpretive comments on dynamics were awkward to make.

It would be a mistake, however, to imagine that the middle-class, and often white, South African psychoanalytic practitioners were any less awkwardly placed than the visiting psychoanalysts. For some, this was a first exposure to kinds of clinical and community work with trauma from which their class, and therefore privilege, had protected them. Uneasily poised between the "I live here" stance of a native to the land, and awareness of knowing far too little about the "here" in which "I" apparently live, not because of geographical distance, but dissociation, many of my compatriots fell silent, and looked eagerly to those moments at which they might begin to feel more completely "at home." Ironically, this moment would come as they listened to much-anticipated papers to be delivered by psychoanalytic luminaries at last visiting our shores.

In this way, the stage was set for an enactment of a colonial encounter with roots in a deep structure buried in a colonial past. Stripped of the complexity and nuance of its surface negotiations, the structure that seemed to drive the enactment could be stated in this way: it involved a rupture of a geographical boundary by a colonizing group with access to mobility, money and knowledge entering with the intention of fertilizing, educating and forever changing the inhabitants they found. In addition to this primal encounter with the indigenous was the role of settlers, those who were once invaders, but having "settled," with all the ambivalence of "settling for" that the phrase implies, found themselves between this "home" and that "home" from which they traced a genealogy.

There were two triggers around which the conference's equilibrium seemed finally to shatter. For an audience that could not be assumed to be proficient in psychoanalytic theory, visiting analysts defaulted on occasion to detailed explanation of basic concepts such as "unconscious" or "transference." While this was clearly intended to demystify psychoanalytic jargon for many in the audience with experience as mental health practitioners but no background of reading psychoanalytic texts, for some this felt like an intolerable dumbing down, as if the years of diasporic reading, study and casework, bravely and unfalteringly undertaken despite absence of elders, was not being acknowledged. Uneasiness and irritation led to an eruption. With previously absent parents engaged at last, the stage was set for ruthlessness. One South African delegate passionately demanded, "Why offer us a bottle when we're ready for solids?" Ivey astutely points out that the mother/baby metaphor was bound to surface in a group collectively, albeit often unconsciously, trying to metabolize an abandonment of children by parents in the face of the horrors of the apartheid regime (Ivey, 1998).

The second rupture spoke to another part of the colonial situation, that in which the trauma itself was residing. Trauma, constantly invoked throughout the conference, became embodied in the sudden cries of a woman overcome with her feelings about her traumatic experience during an exile made necessary by apartheid. She left the room and several people followed her to offer what comfort they could. Her agitation pierced the fabric of that day, breaking up the illusion that we could reflect on our situation without surrendering to its affective resonance for everyone in the hall. It was an essential rupture.

As a local delegate to this conference, and a South African discussant of a visiting psychoanalyst's paper, I was more than simply a witness. I was aware of the effort and care taken to make this an inclusive event, and to draw attention to the rich ways in which the mental health community had risen to the challenges of apartheid and post-apartheid trauma. As an active member of local psychoanalytic groups, I was aware, too, of the broad strokes of our foundational psychoanalytic knowledge. When agitation broke through the surface of scholarly debate, I deeply admired the way in which the rupture was immediately addressed and contained. Our theory and practice saved the day. The events themselves now offer a unique case study of a colonial situation and to think through what its decolonization might entail as we move forward.

The pivot on which the rupture turned was locked into place by ambivalent dependency. It seemed that local delegates could speak only of themselves and their desire for nourishment from shores beyond themselves. International delegates spoke not of themselves, but of what was assumed to be universally true. While local delegates had confidence to speak of themselves, they demurred and became bashful at the thought of wrestling with an internationally accepted body of psychoanalytic wisdoms. And what would it have meant for international delegates to argue with each other about those wisdoms in front of the "children"?

This formulation does carry the potential to point to a route beyond the colonial, entailing simply this: whether we are "local" or "international," we need to preserve a balance between speaking for ourselves, the particularity of contexts, and the shape of the psychoanalytic canon. Psychoanalytic "truths" have always been shaped in the oscillation between theoretical tenet and illustrative case. Coloniality rests in the "case" being located geographically in a diaspora, with "truth" centrally generated being used to explicate it. To decolonize requires both theory and case to be freed from constraining geographies of knowledge.

The Changes conference is still mentioned from time to time by those who attended, or heard about it from others, as memorable, particularly for the way in which it created pain for those who felt misunderstood or unacknowledged, and for those who felt shame in having been caught up in what seemed like a powerful enactment of envy in the face of a generous gesture of connection. That it became an attack on linking few would dispute (Bion, 1959; Ivey, 1998; Samuels, personal communication, 2017). Decades later, and through a decolonizing lens, the rupture and its repair seems an inevitable outcome of a colonial situation being ruthlessly challenged. Collective survival of the collision has been critical to the ways in which we have been able to move forward since.

It is significant that a 2016 psychoanalytic conference, entitled "Couch and Country," held in Cape Town under the auspices of the South African

Psychoanalytic Confederation, and richly representing psychoanalytic theory and practice in South Africa, was a tribute to a diasporic survival, and a powerful assertion of independence from colonial tethers. Its lively debates, frank sharing of opinion on difficult topics, and celebration of work in diverse settings is an important step towards decoloniality. The two conferences are bookends marking a period of substantial shift in psychoanalytic identity and authority, a progress towards coming of age. They mark continuity, in the rich textures of our work, and the kinds of problems that preoccupy us all. They also mark a claim to an autonomous and busy life, independent of central authority. The rupture and repair of the 1998 conference, and its complicated fertilization of the local by the international, was a part of a wrestle with coloniality that made the success of the 2016 event possible. The colonial continues to insert itself as a persistent dynamic, however, and it is to some of these tenacious filaments that I now turn.

Centre and periphery

The crude terms of coloniality assume centres and peripheries. Centres are seats of authority and power; this is sometimes manifest as invading armies or economic might, and sometimes as having rights to adjudicating knowledge hierarchies. Coloniality sets up a relationship of dependence. Again crudely: colonizers bring "civilization," or economic opportunity, or knowledge, in exchange for labour, raw materials, and for some of those colonized, potential membership, under negotiated terms, of a colonized elite. Colonial situations require the ongoing presence of both the colonized and the colonizers; erasure of either side disrupts the terms of coloniality. To decolonize entails the need to destabilize the colonial terms of negotiation, to interrogate the relationship of centre to periphery, to assert the legitimacy of local knowledges, and to work towards undoing dependence on both sides. In Winnicott's terms, decolonization means giving up the exchange of projection that object relating implies. It also means giving up unconscious dependence in favour of the losses and gains of object usage, in which mutual recognition and relative independence are rooted.

From its inception, psychoanalysis has had a history of claiming centralized authority, the legitimacy of which is ratified through hierarchies of certified training, and more informally through kinship networks in which transfer of knowledge and skill might be traced through analyses and supervisions, to the founding fathers. The SAPT was making a bold assertion of intent in wanting to reconnect South Africa to this kinship. It was offering access to this genealogy, and through it to membership of the centre. This remains a project, and centrally recognized psychoanalytic training is now available to South Africans wishing to pursue it. However, massification of the centre does not eliminate peripheries. As the centre grows, so too do peripheries proliferate.

There are a number of ways in which the centre/periphery dynamic in psychoanalysis is being destabilized, and these all contribute to undoing a colonial deep structure. Most importantly, what we are "liable to inherit" is no longer a single strand of DNA. The psychoanalytic centre contains a variety of schools, each laying claim to being psychoanalytic, and this complicates lines of kinship and patronage. So, for example, South African psychoanalytic practitioners have formal and informal links with a variety of international organizations, including Jungian, Freudian, object relations, Kleinian, self and relational groups. Debate locally between schools, joint meetings and collective conferences produce significant dissemination of ideas across schools, all of which dismantle the notion that there is a single theoretical line to be handed down through apprenticeship and study of classical texts.

Along with the spread of psychoanalytic schools, and the constant revisions within each of both foundational Freudian theory and their own basic stance, is a publishing industry that quickly disseminates knowledge through channels independent of tribal membership. The psychoanalytic world is no longer dependent on a handful of journals watched vigilantly by gatekeeping editors. This democratization of knowledge has been one conduit through which new developments in neuroscience and social and political theory have become significant influences on psychoanalytic theory-building.

There have also been significant attempts in some quarters to give voice to peripheries through efforts of editorial boards and conference organizers. The hegemony of northern hemisphere seniors dominating plenary panels, and through this setting up knowledge cycles of what constitutes legitimate writing, thinking and speaking, has made way for challenges to central lines of authority. Where this is partial, it is the result of the repetition at times of the old colonial fault line, in which those in diasporas continue to place themselves as exotic – or at best hybrid – and not builders of "universal" theory that might apply equally at "home" and "abroad." To the extent that leading-edge theorists in psychoanalysis persist in using universalizing language that fails to address the race, class and gender specificity of every case, there will continue to be a split between a theoretical centre and an exceptionalist periphery, a celebration of the exotic other that proves the rule (Chakrabarty, 1998; Long, 2016a, 2017b).

Revisiting psychoanalytic universals: the "primitive"

In the previous section, I argued that the colonial impulse in psychoanalysis rests partly in lines of authority running from a commanding centre to peripheries. Peripheries are conceived in various ways: as repositories of difference to be studied; as opportunities for expansion and potential exploitation through the spreading of the psychoanalytic word; through a "civilizing mission" in which the colonial subject is "educable" and can be "brought in line" with international standards; or through an ideology imbued with liberal humanism, which extends a helping hand to groups of people seen as being in need. Each of these manifestations is a trope ubiquitous in colonial histories. Recognizing the colonial impulse in them all should not obviate against understanding the complexity of each, or the variation in their effects.

Plurality of voice, wide dissemination of central debates, and generous opportunities to participate in international conferences, seminars and colloquia have significantly altered a colonial situation with central ownership of knowledge and power. Regardless of this decentring, what are we "liable to inherit" by reading psychoanalysis and employing its methods? It is to this question that my argument now turns.

Psychoanalysis has many parts and formidable strengths, not least of which is its capacity to critique its own methods and conclusions. Its broad influence as a philosophy of mind, and responsiveness to demand for both theoretical and technical change, has ensured its enduring legacy. The argument that follows concerns the ways in which psychoanalytic theory has played a part in creating the colonial subject. This in turn leads to a repetition of a colonial situation in which those colonized find themselves invisible, simplified, made childish, or "recognized" only through what their colonizers allow them to become. To unravel the depths of this would be a major undertaking beyond the scope of this chapter, but it is incisively tackled in the work of Brickman (2003), Hook (2013), Hook and Truscott (2013), Khanna (2003), Layton et al. (2006) and many others. Here, I will take up two pivotal psychoanalytic concepts only: the primitive, and gendered colonial subjectivity.

As Hook and Truscott (2013) point out, Freud's model of mind accomplished the extraordinary feat of insisting on the primitive as everywhere, in everyone, as a source of impulse and energy, an immediacy of instinct untrammelled by social restrictions. Nonetheless, its embeddedness in psychoanalytic theory needs to be a point of interrogation in the decolonial discussion. It was central to the success of colonial power, and carries often ill-defined ideas of what it is to be "civilized" into the heart of psychoanalytic theory.

Overlapping with British colonialism at its height, evolutionary theory, capturing and then proliferating the idea of higher and lower life forms, "primitive" and civilized races, was strongly implicated in the political, economic and social policies of British colonial practice because it provided a perfect rationalization for the assertion that colonizers were superior to those colonized. There was, of course, a fear of backsliding, of settlers "going native" through exposure to indigenous people's way of life. This in turn became the rationalization for policing the boundary between groups, in order to minimize the opportunity for social and sexual contact (Swartz, 1995; Truscott, 2013). The fear of contamination of the civilized by the "primitive" had an additional layer. By casting indigenous groups in colonized countries as "primitive," they instantly became "knowable" either as "childish" or "simple"; further enquiry into their humanity was unnecessary. Moreover, thinking of colonized people as "primitive" allowed the traumatic effects of colonialism to be disregarded. The lunatic asylum casebooks of Cape Colony record with dismal regularity that the causes of a black patient's episodes of insanity were "unknown." This failure to engage with lunatic asylum inmates as suffering individuals is one consequence of seeing their mentality as too "primitive," too childish or too deviant to warrant careful investigation (Swartz, 2015).

It was a form of defensive reductionism that continues to operate whenever otherness becomes conflated with being simply one characteristic: "black," or "gay," or "disabled."

The term "primitive," applied to thinking in particular, has a long and consequential history in all the social sciences (Samuels, 2015; Swartz, 2015). It unfolds as one pole of the description that draws a line from "savage" to "civilized," with the "primitive" being associated with magical thinking and superstition (Freud, 1913). Taking assumption as fact over decades, colonial psychiatry shaped its practices to obscure the suffering of colonized peoples, and justified this on the grounds that "natives" lacked the capacity to have "higher forms" of mental illness, such as depression (Carothers, 1948). This is one way in which trauma was permitted and obscured in colonial societies (Swartz, 2015, pp. 183–205).

Brickman's authoritative reading of the "primitive" in psychoanalytic theory demonstrates the ways in which it was shot through with evolutionary theory that ranked groups according to their cultural and mental sophistication (Brickman, 2003). It is taken further by embedding the idea that every individual, from infancy to adulthood, recapitulates this evolutionary scale. As she notes:

> In the very act of bridging the great divide between civilized and primitive as seen by colonial anthropology, by enlisting the figure of the primitive to represent a universal stratum of the mind, Freud placed this figure at the beginning and/or in the unconscious of a developmentally ordered model of the mind, representing the primitive as both constituting, yet partially excluded from, modern civilized subjectivity.
>
> (Brickman, 2003, p. 245)

Brickman argues convincingly that the use of the term "primitive" in psychoanalytic theory is irrevocably tied to histories of race, and the designation of colonized races as "primitive." She suggests that in this way, even a concept such as regression, entailing a return to the past and to infantile emotional states, necessarily conjures a civilized present, and further that this "civilization" is associated with the kinds of white heteronormativity that have so often been assumed, without careful interrogation. In her view, Freud, "by casting difference as deviation and accounting for anomaly by regression, thereby consigning difference to the past . . . insured that psychoanalysis would conflate racial/cultural difference with pathology and see both as evolutionarily and developmentally prior to white western norms" (Brickman, 2003, p. 255).

According to Brickman, therefore, the "primitive" is a central facet of psychoanalytic theory, throned in the significance given to instinctual life or primary process thinking, and the embeddedness of both concepts in the construction of colonized subjectivities. It has a further coronation through the "developmental tilt" of post-Freudian psychoanalytic theory (Mitchell, 1984, p. 477). As Stephen Mitchell's brilliant paper argued, theory-building in psychoanalysis after Freud found the earliest years of infancy an uncolonized territory in which to place a flag, without crossing swords with the law of the father, thus welding the "primitive" indelibly into states of high arousal in infancy and ruthless struggle towards selfhood.

Apart from its baggage in colonial racism, there are two immediate arguments to be made in favour of problematizing the idea of the "primitive" across schools of psychoanalytic thought; in time, there may be more. First, infant research has fundamentally interrupted the possibility of regarding infancy as a time during which processing of information is "primitive" (Beebe and Lachmann, 2013; Stern, 1985). Moreover, systems of mutual regulation between infants and caregivers carry complex signalling long before the establishment of verbal language. The implications of being aware of this non-symbolic realm for therapeutic dyads is explicated in Knoblauch (2017). As he points out:

> Currently our analytic culture still overprivileges cognitive imagining as the ideal for emotional-self control. This kind of privileging too often makes the body either invisible or potentially "primitive," needing to be contained rather than received as a source of credible and useful meanings. This cultural bias can erase, or at least make opaque, the capacity of the analyst to recognize and make use of his own vulnerability for its therapeutic value.
>
> (Knoblauch, 2017, p. 306)

To continue to think of states of regression to infancy as a movement backwards into more and more "primitive" states of being therefore makes sense no longer.

Second, arguing for a hierarchy of defences, from the "primitive" to the mature, is complicated by ways in which we now take for granted the multiplicity of selfhood. This includes, but is not confined to, the effects of dissociation on conscious awareness. Dissociation describes one form of multilayered consciousness, and is defensive against overwhelming or painful affect states. Other forms of multiplicity, with the movement in and out of "selves," are an everyday part of communication between people (Bromberg, 2013; Brothers, 2014; Danielian and Gianotti, 2012). Each self-state will be associated with a range of defences, depending on its affective colouring, links to particular patterns of attachment, and levels of threat or security. Dyadic communication therefore is likely to involve hierarchies of defence attached to multiple self-states, rather than a single one.

Similarly, to cast protesting crowds as being in the sway of a single – and "primitive" or irrational – state of mind does less than justice to the multiple layers of thinking that might be taking place from moment to moment in and between individuals.

So, recasting the ways in which the term "primitive" is used in psychoanalysis has the potential to undo a historical link to the figure of the "primitive" that has endured from late nineteenth- and early twentieth-century anthropology, to assert fluidity and multiplicity in the place of rigid sets of defences, and to refuse the idea of infant perception and affectivity as either crude or solipsistic. Most importantly, it undoes an implicit hierarchy; after all, wherever the "primitive" is identified, a "mature" or "civilized" mind has made that judgement, with all the machinations of power that implies.

In evaluating the provenance of the "primitive" in psychoanalytic theory, it is useful to compare it to ruthlessness, its conceptual cousin. The "primitive" is defined partly by invoking "maturity" as an opposite; "ruthlessness" – single-mindedness – might mature into "ruth," which involves a capacity to mind the minds of others. Following Winnicott, the explorations in this book have insisted on ruthlessness as an assertion of selfhood, a place from which to speak that is untrammelled by compliance, the compromise of the needs of the self to those of another. To be ruthless is to insist on recognition; if there is to be mutuality, ruthlessness is a necessary precursor. Further, ruthless states of mind are the origin of the spontaneous gesture, the source of creativity. In the sense that the true self, and the source of ruthlessness, precedes compliance, and therefore entry into the social, it might be regarded as original. It is problematic, however, to suggest either that this is "primitive" or that regression is the route to discovery of the true self. Pursuit of authenticity, perhaps a better description of true self, entails not a return to an unspoiled (and "primitive") state of innocence, but to a less compromised negotiation between self and other constantly being remade through the course of development. It requires a degree of ruthlessness to show up authentically, and this grows rather than diminishes with widening awareness of competing needs between self and others.

Revisiting psychoanalytic universals: the place of gender

Colonialism was made possible by a world view that created indigenous peoples as susceptible to being ruled; in other words, it is predicated on a basic assumption that the "civilized" and the rational, as qualities, endow some with rights over those deemed "uncivilized" or irrational. It is this set of assumptions that animated psychoanalytic theory too, a model in which the instinctive and the "primitive" must of necessity bow to the reasonable and the mature for the sake of social order. There is a second layer of assumption in this narrative: in colonialism, it is the figure of the white man who is "reasonable"; women, by contrast, are to be protected from danger. These dangers come from without, in the form of attack on their vulnerable bodies, and from within, in the form of feminine irrationality and a predisposition to flights of fancy. Colonialism thus naturalized white male dominance in particular, and cast binary gender roles as too obvious to warrant explanation.

Work undoing psychoanalytic theory's history of assuming heterosexuality and gender binaries as natural and normal is well under way. There is a substantial literature on the gender and psychoanalysis that tackles the ways in which it bolsters patriarchal assumptions, reinforces the gendering of social roles, and posits heterosexuality as a norm, against which all other forms of sexual expression are regarded as deviant (see Benjamin, 1998; Burkhalter, 2015; Cooper, 2003; Corbett, 2009; Davies, 2003; Dimen and Goldner, 2005; Gentile, 2015; Mitchell, 2000). Just as a decolonial project must worry about the use of the term "primitive," so too must it worry about the naturalized lines of power and passivity that comes packaged with colonial (and psychoanalytic) structuring of gendered subjectivity. This gendering, and the ways in which colonialism shaped trajectories through the oedipal, is of significance in thinking through the decolonization of psychoanalysis in particular.

Colonial subjects have a complicated history in relation to being gendered (Abrahams, 1996; Boonzaier, 2017; McClintock, 1995). On the one hand, the threat of "savage" races was frequently expressed in their men being seen as hypersexualized, and as a result a sexual threat to colonizer women positioned as vulnerable (Swartz, 2015). This in turn gave colonizing men permission to "protect" their women specifically against the possibility of sexual assault (Bergner, 1995; Sharpe, 1991). In the 1913 De Villiers *Report of the Commission Appointed to Enquire into Assaults on Women*, a remarkable document laying out colonial attitudes towards sexuality and race, this is extended to recommendations regarding precautions that need to be taken by white women to protect themselves against sexual assault. These include suggesting that "women should not wander about alone," that "daughters of the house should have as little as possible" to do with black male servants, and that "precautions should be taken properly to secure the doors and windows of the room in which women sleep, and in undressing they should take care that the blinds are carefully drawn" (De Villiers, 1913, pp. 28–29). The assumption here of white women as sexually alluring, as well as unmindful of the dangers in which they place themselves, gives the permission for white men not only to protect, but to think for them too. The rhetoric is even more vehement with respect to the employment of black men as caregivers for children. In a narrative that describes black men as initiating young girls of their community into sexual play, two settler colonial prohibitions are foregrounded: public and accepted pleasure in sexual activity, and the education of girls into its practice.

The collapse of "primitive" into the category "childish" complicated the narrative of the dangerous sexuality, by rendering the colonial subject as simultaneously a sexual threat *and* in need of supervision and education, a kind of timeless latency life that, in its passivity, had more to do with the psychoanalytic feminine than with a collision between two patriarchal systems. It is no mistake that many labouring men in colonial systems were referred to as "boys." The Commission talks, for example, about the "depravity engendered amongst the natives by contact with the evils of civilization," such as liquor, criminal activity and prostitution (De Villiers, 1913, p. 21). This reading of the "primitive" positions white men as protecting the innocence of a "pure" and unspoiled society uncorrupted by collision with the demands of a higher order of moral demand and constraint.

In this narrative, black male colonial subjects were characterized as both sexual and childishly innocent, and black female colonial subjects were seen as alluring in their exotic otherness, ravishing and susceptible to being ravished (by their colonizers) outside of the boundaries of traditional family life. This then became embodied in their sexual exploitation, taking place outside of the monogamy and sexual abstemiousness written into "civilized" colonizer family mores. Colonial men, in this narrative, were lured away from lawfulness and rationality, and behaved in ways that enacted the lawless sexuality they saw as belonging to the "primitive" populations they were exploiting. It all took place in the shadows, and was far from "civilized" (Hall, 2002; Levine, 2004; Martens, 2002; Phillips, 2009; Veracini, 2010).

It is unsurprising, given the world of splitting, projection and consequent double standards that infected colonial worlds, that anxiety about miscegenation was never far from the surface (Bland, 2005; Brah and Coombes, 2005; Stoler, 2010). Fear of racial degeneration through the reproduction of colonial subjects of "mixed" racial identities was tied up with backsliding down an evolutionary hierarchy, of becoming racially polluted or tainted through sexual liaisons across racial boundaries (Oppenheim, 1991; Stoler, 2010; Swartz, 1995). The boundaries were, however, constantly confirmed in the breach, either in fantasy (for example, the fear of colonized subjects taking advantage of vulnerable colonizer women) or in actuality (for example, the women in colonized populations being used for the "necessary" release of sexual frustration of unmarried colonizer men). The breach of boundaries also expressed the ubiquity of perverse sexuality, which in turned led to a redoubling of effort to maintain "purity."

Freud insisted that the "primitive" is an enduring part of human existence, and cannot be split off and located in the bodies and lives of the colonial or cultural other. The "primitive" would become "mature" through development. Similarly, he insisted on the sexual as being a part of human existence from infancy, beginning as wayward and perverse, and being tamed into moderation through "appropriate" object choice in adulthood. Publicly proscribed were promiscuity, and forms of "perverse" sexuality such as homosexuality and all sexual contact with children. Prescribed was a model of monocultural nuclear family life, boundaried in such a way that the longings, fears and competition of the children born to the heterosexual couple might be safely traversed, and leave intact the father's idealizable authority.

Proscriptions and prescriptions were thrown into stark relief by the colonial situation, which endlessly reproduced anxiety about deviating from a model of heterosexuality confined to the boundaries of a nuclear family. Particular to colonial lists of the publicly forbidden, along with various forms of perversity, promiscuity, homosexuality and child sexual abuse, was sexual intimacy across racial boundaries. Respectability, rigidly policed, became a charm against the danger of "going native." At the same time, disavowed sexual contact with colonial subjects, with all its connotations of taboo desire, was a threat to respectability, and reinforced the need to defend rigidly its reliance on gendered, generational and racial binaries. The colonial situation, with its demotion of subjects to perpetual childhood by authoritarian regimes, its sexualization of those deemed to be children in thought and deed, and the anxiety-driven shoring up of boundaries along with insistence on binaries, constellated a split universe (Truscott, 2013). In one, the colonizer world, there was a path through the unconscious terrors of the oedipal. In the other, the world of the colonial subject, there was transgression and castration. In other words, there was no path into adult sexuality that did not involve violence.

This suggests that the way through to decolonizing will therefore include undoing gender and sexuality binaries that coercively obscured the complexity of being a sexual actor in the colonial situation at the same as insisting on forms of sexual embodiment that gave legitimacy to the colonizing regime. As Morgensen suggests:

> Anticolonial feminist and queer accounts show that colonisation's sexual and gendered methods are inventive, not foreordained; and that liberation will follow disturbing all that colonisation taught, so that distinctive ways of life might be recalled or imagined. Such accounts position "gender" and "sexuality" alongside "race" and "nation" as analytical categories that are freed from any universal referent, in that they designate power-laden arenas of contested knowledge and embodied practice that call for critical and creative engagement.
>
> (Morgensen, 2012, p. 5)

I am suggesting here that anxieties ubiquitous in the colonial situation would have fed into the heteronormative orthodoxy of psychoanalytic theory, through exactly the route that also shaped its foundational embrace of the notion of "primitive" mental life. Both are rooted in projects of exploration and conquest that mapped the exotic, observed otherness, and used both to define normality, while erasing the infinite variability of subject formation. It makes sense, then, that the decolonial subject must argue with and refuse the kinds of respectable monocultural nuclear family life from which he or she was consciously and unconsciously barred in the colonial situation by child status, and by assumptions of otherness. The #RhodesMustFall and #FeesMustFall movements on South African campuses argued forcefully and effectively that decolonial political movements will inevitably fall short without the insertion of LGBTQI perspectives and rights into their centre.

The decolonial subject will – must – refuse race and gender either as biological givens or as social constructions inexorably bolstered by the trappings of ideology. To conceive of both race and gender as multiple, and further as mutually shaping, frees individual development from the shackles of compulsory membership of either, and radically expands possibilities of individual choice. Psychoanalytic theory, decolonized along these lines, may therefore conceive of passage through oedipal conflict as the place in which an individual tussles with relational, social and political demands, instead of carrying through an instinctually driven or ideologically prescriptive unconscious agenda with a constricted ending. The relational reworking of the oedipal drama stresses also the mutuality of struggles around difference, exclusion and competition, and the love affair itself is a welcome antidote to the rather grim biologically driven fate of the Freudian oedipal child, who must lose, and lose utterly, to the parental couple (Benjamin, 2002; Cooper, 2003; Davies, 2003; Swartz, 2007a).

One example will illustrate the ways in which identity formation during the oedipal struggle might be expressed as a complicating of race and gender binaries. In Adrienne Rich's dialogue with her father in "Sources," she grapples with the intricacy and contradictions of both her gender identity and her Jewish heritage (Rich, 1986). She describes what it means to have been treated as she imagines a son might have been, a scholar, an arguer through text. At the same time, born into a world in which being Jewish confers on her and her family an identity of outsider, there is an experience of being both foreign or alien, and yet having lost the meaning of belonging "elsewhere" through the shaping forces of assimilation. What has been lost through the accommodation to a new "home" is an identification – a kinship – with Jews persecuted precisely through marking and stigmatizing their difference from those with political power. She finds herself placed at intersections that undo binaries at every turn, born into a deracinated Jewish identity, foreign and assimilated, and being offered the position of son to a father who taught her to read and write without the soothing incantation of prayer.

For Rich, then, overthrowing her father brings her into possession of all that he has disavowed; by being chosen as the son, the heir, she inherits not only the books, the ability to argue, to read and write, but also the content of his unconscious, his Other. There is no resolution; he lives on as her constant companion, as she reaches for everything he is not.

Conclusion

I have argued in this chapter that the decolonization of psychoanalysis has two parts. One involves the complicated task of understanding the ways in which psychoanalytic theory was influenced historically by the colonial situation in fundamental ways. The historical analysis provides a lens through which versions of coloniality continue to shape ways in which subjectivity is formed within social, political, class and cultural constraints. This part of the argument suggests that for psychoanalytic theory to be decolonized, it needs to replace the coercions of apparent "universals" with the infinite choice of the particular, the variable, the multiple routes to spontaneity and freedom. The second part of the argument concerns practices of transmitting psychoanalytic DNA from centre to periphery, parent to child. This involves quarrelling with authorities guarding the gates of psychoanalytic theory, all those with the power to decide what constitutes legitimate psychoanalytic knowledge, and will of necessity involve interrogation of licensing bodies, editorial boards and conference committees, everywhere. There is rich evidence that the decolonizing project is flourishing: as I hope I have shown, disentangling psychoanalysis from its coloniality, both in its theoretical underpinnings and its relationship to central authority, is producing rich rewards. The ruthlessness of the project, and surviving the quarrels wherever they occur, has "put the brakes on" fantasies about the infinite wisdoms those in peripheries have forced those in the centre to carry (Winnicott, 2002, p. 153). It has also produced a challenge to all those living in psychoanalytic diasporas to "put the brakes on" fantasies of their voicelessness. Coming up against central authority and dismantling some of its restricting ways demands new forms of negotiation. As Winnicott's exploration of ruthlessness demonstrates, after the collision, and survival, comes a settling with all the compromises that holding multiplicity entails. For those in psychoanalytic diasporas, this entails giving up on deferral of authority to others, and the responsibility of finding new and appropriate forms of agency.

In settler colonies, being far from the mother country ("home") produced anxiety in colonizers about being irrevocably damaged by strangeness and estrangement – anxiety about "going native," being driven mad by the sun, failing to maintain "civilized" standards. The defence against these anxieties was to try as far as possible to recreate "home" in the colonial setting. This included mimicry of every form of governance, daily routine, building, school curriculum and social convention in the colony. At times, this produced clubs, schools, hospitals and rules that were exaggerated versions of those at "home." Holding nostalgia, and the possibility of feeling "at home" in places made strange by the colonizing gaze, these institutions of settler colonies rigidly enforced ways of living that were obdurate in their refusal to mould themselves to the invitations and challenges of local contexts.

There have been times, in this South African psychoanalytic diaspora, that some have been tempted into the same entrapping impulse – to replicate institutions, forms of teaching and training, that, like transitional objects, will reassure that the parenting which is longed for is continuous. It is a colonial – diasporic – worry about survival and rescue from anxious endurance of separation.

With decolonizing in mind, the task going forward is clear. It is neither appropriate nor practical to replicate the centre's rich proliferations of psychoanalytic training in a context with mental health resources failing to meet even the most basic aid to those urgently in need. At the same time, local practitioners have been extraordinarily inventive in finding ways to shape practice to demand, improvising and producing a bespoke psychoanalytic reflectiveness that is contextually sensitive and always ready to change its rules of operation. Finally, there is the task of negotiating authority. This is not to reject, discredit or displace authorities with international legitimacy, but to find a place at the table and to speak not only of colonial exoticism, but accumulated experience with theoretical and practical fundamentals, in ways that will complicate naturalized assumptions and add substantively to a psychoanalytic future.

This exploration of the decolonial project in psychoanalysis has been about parents and children, acquiring personhood, and holding on to the possibility of originality. It is also about hoping that the spontaneous gesture will be received. It is about rebellion against authority, and distinguishing oneself as both independent and being authoritative in that independence. Winnicott, whose revisions of Freud and Klein were ruthless, and insisted on his originality, has much to contribute to thinking through the complexity of the issues at hand. Most of all, he presented his audience with a way forward, beyond defensive isolation, beyond compliance and mimicry. It is with this that I would like to end the argument.

Winnicott's essential optimism about the capacity of parents and children to muddle through collisions and misrecognitions and to survive is invested in the idea that many parents are "good enough," and that through a series of adaptations on both sides, all will be well. The colonial situation in general cannot be described in this way – the parents were never "good enough"; they were cruel and even murderous, and disavowed the humanity of their subjects. This was not the case with psychoanalytic parenting, although it has always taken on the prejudices, blind spots and cultural coloring of its times. From time to time, its gaze distorted the subject in view. Sometimes its methods built in corrections to these distortions over time. The point is not the distortion, but the act of sight, and what it allows. Moreover, psychoanalysis has faced many searching critiques from theorists and practitioners operating in and out of its mainstream conventions and survived. To paraphrase Winnicott, of this South African diaspora, it might be said, "When we looked, we were seen, so we exist" (indeed we were created by this exchange of sight). "We can now afford to look and see" (Winnicott, 1971, p. 134).

References

Abrahams, Y. (1996). Disempowered to consent: Sara Bartman and Khoisan slavery in the nineteenth-century Cape colony and Britain. *South African Historical Journal*, *35*(1), 89–114.

Beebe, B. and Lachmann, F. M. (2013). *Infant research and adult treatment: Co-constructing interactions*. Routledge.

Benjamin, J. (1998). *Like subjects, love objects: Essays on recognition and sexual difference*. Yale University Press.

Benjamin, J. (2002). The question of sexual difference. *Feminism and Psychology*, *12*, 39–43.

Bergner, G. (1995). Who is that masked woman? Or, the role of gender in Fanon's *Black Skin, White Masks*. *Publications of the Modern Language Association of America*, *110*(1), 75–88.

Bion, W. (1959). Attacks on linking. *The International Journal of Psycho-Analysis*, *40*, 308–315.

Bland, L. (2005). White women and men of colour: Miscegenation fears in Britain after the Great War. *Gender & History*, *17*(1), 29–61.

Boonzaier, F. (2017). The life and death of Anene Booysen: Colonial discourse, gender-based violence and media representations. *South African Journal of Psychology*, *47*(4), 470–481.

Brah, A. and Coombes, A. (Eds.) (2005). *Hybridity and its discontents: Politics, science, culture*. Routledge.

Brickman, C. (2003). *Aboriginal populations in the mind: Race and primitivity in psychoanalysis*. Columbia University Press.

Bromberg, P. M. (2013). *Awakening the dreamer: Clinical journeys*. Routledge.

Brothers, D. (2014). Traumatic attachments: Intergenerational trauma, dissociation, and the analytic relationship. *International Journal of Psychoanalytic Self Psychology*, *9*(1), 3–15.

Burkhalter, T. (2015). Imagining masculinities through an exilic consciousness. *Studies in Gender and Sexuality*, *16*(4), 290–303.

Carothers, J. C. (1948). A study of mental derangement in Africans, and an attempt to explain its peculiarities, more especially in relation to the African attitude to life. *Psychiatry*, *11*(1), 47–86.

Chakrabarty, D. (1998). Minority histories, subaltern pasts. *Scrutiny2*, *3*(1), 4–15.
Cooper, S. H. (2003). You say oedipal, I say postoedipal: A consideration of desire and hostility in the analytic relationship. *Psychoanalytic Dialogues*, *13*(1), 41–63.
Corbett, K. (2009). Boyhood femininity, gender identity disorder, masculine presuppositions, and the anxiety of regulation. *Psychoanalytic Dialogues*, *19*(4), 353–370.
Danielian, J. and Gianotti, P. (2012). *Listening with purpose: Entry points into shame and narcissistic vulnerability*. Jason Aronson.
Davies, J. M. (2003). Falling in love with love: Oedipal and postoedipal manifestations of idealization, mourning, and erotic masochism. *Psychoanalytic Dialogues*, *13*(1), 1–27.
De Villiers (2013). *Report of the Commission Appointed to Enquire into Assaults on Women*. U.G. 39-'13.
Dimen, M. and Goldner, V. (2005). Gender and sexuality. In E. S. Person, A. M. Cooper and G. O. Gabbard (Eds.), *The American Psychiatric Publishing textbook of psychoanalysis* (pp. 93–114). American Psychiatric Publishing.
Dubow, S. (1993). Wulf Sachs's *Black Hamlet*: A case of "psychic vivisection"? *African Affairs*, *92*(369), 519–556.
Dubow, S. (1995). *Scientific racism in modern South Africa*. Cambridge University Press.
Freud, S. (1913). *Totem and taboo: The standard edition of the complete psychological works of Sigmund Freud* (Vol. 13), trans. J. Strachey. Hogarth Press.
Gentile, J. (2015). On having no thoughts: Freedom and feminine space. *Psychoanalytic Perspectives*, *12*(3), 227–251.
Greenlees, T. D. (1895). Insanity among the natives of South Africa. *The British Journal of Psychiatry*, *41*(172), 71–78.
Hall, C. (2002). *Civilising subjects: Metropole and colony in the English imagination 1830–1867*. University of Chicago Press.
Hayes, G. (2008). A history of psychoanalysis in South Africa. *Interiors*, 182–189.
Hook, D. (2013). *(Post) apartheid conditions: Psychoanalysis and social formation*. Springer.
Hook, D. and Truscott, R. (2013). Fanonian ambivalence: On psychoanalysis and postcolonial critique. *Journal of Theoretical and Philosophical Psychology*, *33*(3), 155–169.
Ivey, G. (1998). Pure gold or therapeutic alloy? Some issues raised by the conference "Change: Psychoanalytic perspectives." Psychology in Society (PINS), *23*, 52–57.
Kagee, A. (2006). Where is the evidence in South African clinical psychology? *South African Journal of Psychology*, *36*(2), 233–248.
Khanna, R. (2003). *Dark continents: Psychoanalysis and colonialism*. Duke University Press.
Knoblauch, S. H. (2017). The fluidity of emotions and clinical vulnerability: A field of rhythmic tensions. *Psychoanalytic Perspectives*, *14*(3), 283–308.
Layton, L., Hollander, N. C. and Gutwill, S. (Eds.) (2006). *Psychoanalysis, class and politics: Encounters in the clinical setting*. Routledge.
Levine, P. (2004). *Gender and empire*. Oxford University Press.
Long, W. (2016a). *A history of "relevance" in psychology*. Palgrave Macmillan.
Long, W. (2016b). On the Africanization of psychology. *South African Journal of Psychology*, *46*(4), 429–431.
Long, W. (2017a). Alienation: A new orienting principle for psychotherapists in South Africa. *Psycho-Analytic Psychotherapy in South Africa*, *25*(1), 67–90.
Long, W. (2017b). Essence or experience? A new direction for African psychology. *Theory & Psychology*, *27*(3), 293–312.

Martens, J. C. (2002). Settler homes, manhood and "houseboys": An analysis of Natal's rape scare of 1886. *Journal of Southern African Studies, 28*(2), 379–400.
McClintock, A. (1995). *Imperial leather: Gender, race and sexuality in the colonial context.* Routledge.
McCulloch, J. (1995). *Colonial psychiatry and the African mind.* Cambridge University Press.
Mitchell, S.A. (1984). Object relations theories and the developmental tilt. *Contemporary Psychoanalysis, 20*, 473–499.
Mitchell, J. (2000). *Psychoanalysis and feminism: A radical reassessment of Freudian psychoanalysis.* Basic Books.
Morgensen, S. L. (2012). Theorising gender, sexuality and settler colonialism: An Introduction. *Settler Colonial Studies, 2*(2), 2–22.
Oppenheim, J. (1991). *"Shattered nerves": Doctors, patients, and depression in Victorian England.* Oxford University Press.
Phillips, R. (2009). Settler colonialism and the nuclear family. *The Canadian Geographer/ Le Géographe Canadien, 53*(2), 239–253.
Raphael-Leff, J. (2016). *Psychoanalysis in South Africa.* Retrieved 26 September 2016, from https://karnacology.com/?s=raphael+leff.
Rich, A. (1986). *Your native land, your life.* Norton.
Ruane, I. (2010). Obstacles to the utilisation of psychological resources in a South African township community. *South African Journal of Psychology, 40*(2), 214–225.
Sachs, W. (1937). *Black Hamlet.* Geoffrey Bles.
Samuels, A. (2015). *The political psyche.* Routledge.
Sharpe, J. (1991). The unspeakable limits of rape: Colonial violence and counter-insurgency. *Genders, 10*, 25–46.
Stern, D. N. (1985). *The interpersonal world of the infant: A view from psychoanalysis and developmental psychology.* Karnac.
Stoler, A. L. (2001). Tense and tender ties: The politics of comparison in North American history and (post) colonial studies. *The Journal of American History, 88*(3), 829–865.
Stoler, A. L. (2010). *Carnal knowledge and imperial power: Race and the intimate in colonial rule.* University of California Press.
Swartz, R. (2018). Civilisation and colonial education: Natal and Western Australia in the 1860s in comparative perspective. *History of Education, 47*(3), 1–16.
Swartz, S. (1995). Colonizing the insane: Causes of insanity in the Cape, 1891–1920. *History of the Human Sciences, 8*(4), 39–57.
Swartz, S. (2007a). Oedipus matters. *Psychodynamic Practice, 13*(4), 361–373.
Swartz, S. (2007b). Reading psychoanalysis in the diaspora: South African psychoanalytic psychotherapists' struggles with voice. *Psycho-Analytic Psychotherapy in South Africa, 15*(2), 1–18.
Swartz, S. (2015). *Homeless wanderers: Movement and mental illness in the cape colony in the nineteenth century.* UCT Press.
Swartz, S. (2017). Mad Africa. In G. Eghigian (Ed.), *The Routledge history of madness and mental health* (pp. 229–244). Routledge.
Truscott, R. (2013). Obsessional whiteness and the unpaid debt of apartheid. *Social and Personality Psychology Compass, 7*(8), 537–546.
Veracini, L. (2010). *Settler colonialism.* Palgrave Macmillan.
Winnicott, D. W. (1971). *Playing and reality.* Penguin Books.
Winnicott, D. W. (2002). *Through paediatrics to psychoanalysis: Collected papers.* Karnac.

Index

For Product Safety Concerns and Information please contact our EU
representative GPSR@taylorandfrancis.com
Taylor & Francis Verlag GmbH, Kaufingerstraße 24, 80331 München, Germany

www.ingramcontent.com/pod-product-compliance
Ingram Content Group UK Ltd.
Pitfield, Milton Keynes, MK11 3LW, UK
UKHW020137200926
475702UK00005B/791
* 9 7 8 1 1 3 8 3 4 5 4 8 5 *